Neuromodulation in Child and Adolescent Psychiatry

Editors

JONATHAN ESSARY BECKER
CHRISTOPHER TODD MALEY
ELIZABETH K.B. SHULTZ
TODD E. PETERS

CHILD AND ADOLESCENT PSYCHIATRIC CLINICS OF NORTH AMERICA

www.childpsych.theclinics.com

Consulting Editor
TODD E. PETERS

January 2019 • Volume 28 • Number 1

ELSEVIER

1600 John F. Kennedy Boulevard • Suite 1800 • Philadelphia, Pennsylvania, 19103-2899

http://www.theclinics.com

**CHILD AND ADOLESCENT PSYCHIATRIC CLINICS OF NORTH AMERICA Volume 28, Number 1
January 2019 ISSN 1056-4993, ISBN-13: 978-0-323-65461-6**

Editor: Lauren Boyle
Developmental Editor: Kristen Helm

Child and Adolescent Psychiatric Clinics of North America (ISSN 1056-4993) is published quarterly by Elsevier Inc., 360 Park Avenue South, New York, NY 10010-1710. Months of issue are January, April, July, and October. Business and Editorial Offices: 1600 John F. Kennedy Boulevard, Suite 1800, Philadelphia, PA 19103-2899. Periodicals postage paid at New York, NY and additional mailing offices. Subscription prices are $335.00 per year (US individuals), $627.00 per year (US institutions), $100.00 per year (US students), $388.00 per year (Canadian individuals), $762.00 per year (Canadian institutions), $200.00 per year (Canadian students), $446.00 per year (international individuals), $762.00 per year (international institutions), and $200.00 per year (international students). International air speed delivery is included in all *Clinics* subscription prices. All prices are subject to change without notice. **POSTMASTER:** Send address changes to *Child and Adolescent Psychiatric Clinics of North America*, Elsevier Health Sciences Division, Subscription Customer Service, 3251 Riverport Lane, Maryland Heights, MO 63043. **Customer Service: 1-800-654-2452 (U.S. and Canada); 314-447-8871 (outside U.S. and Canada). Fax: 314-447-8029. E-mail:** JournalsCustomer Service-usa@elsevier.com **(for print support) or** journalsonlinesupport-usa@elsevier.com **(for online support).**

Reprints. For copies of 100 or more of articles in this publication, please contact the Commercial Reprints Department, Elsevier Inc., 360 Park Avenue South, New York, New York 10010-1710 Tel.: 212-633-3874; Fax: 212-633-3820, E-mail: reprints@elsevier.com.

Child and Adolescent Psychiatric Clinics of North America is covered in *MEDLINE/PubMed (Index Medicus), ISI, SSCI, Research Alert, Social Search, Current Contents,* and *EMBASE/Excerpta Medica.*

Contributors

CONSULTING EDITOR

TODD E. PETERS, MD, FAPA
Medical Director, Child and Adolescent Services, Chief Medical Information Officer (CMIO), Sheppard Pratt Health System, Sheppard Pratt Physicians PA Clinical Operations Liaison, Baltimore, Maryland

EDITORS

JONATHAN ESSARY BECKER, DO, MS
Assistant Professor of Clinical Psychiatry, Department of Psychiatry and Behavioral Sciences, Director of the Neuromodulation Service, Vanderbilt University Medical School, Vanderbilt Psychiatric Hospital, Nashville, Tennessee, USA

CHRISTOPHER TODD MALEY, MD
Assistant Professor of Clinical Psychiatry, Department of Psychiatry and Behavioral Sciences, Vanderbilt University Medical Center, Vanderbilt Psychiatric Hospital, Nashville, Tennessee, USA

ELIZABETH K.B. SHULTZ, DO
Assistant Professor of Clinical Psychiatry, Department of Psychiatry and Behavioral Sciences, Vanderbilt University Medical Center, Vanderbilt Psychiatric Hospital, Nashville, Tennessee, USA

TODD E. PETERS, MD, FAPA
Medical Director, Child and Adolescent Services, Chief Medical Information Officer (CMIO), Sheppard Pratt Health System, Sheppard Pratt Physicians PA Clinical Operations Liaison, Baltimore, Maryland

AUTHORS

JONATHAN ESSARY BECKER, DO, MS
Assistant Professor of Clinical Psychiatry, Department of Psychiatry and Behavioral Sciences, Director of the Neuromodulation Service, Vanderbilt University Medical School, Vanderbilt Psychiatric Hospital, Nashville, Tennessee, USA

MARGARET M. BENNINGFIELD, MD
Associate Professor, Department of Psychiatry and Behavioral Sciences, Vanderbilt University Medical Center, Nashville, Tennessee, USA

CAREN J. BLACKER, BMBCh, MA
Instructor in Psychiatry, Department of Psychiatry and Psychology, Division of Child and Adolescent Psychiatry, Mayo Clinic, Rochester, Minnesota, USA

DENIZ DORUK CAMSARI, MD
Resident in Psychiatry, Department of Psychiatry and Psychology, Division of Child and Adolescent Psychiatry, Mayo Clinic, Rochester, Minnesota, USA

PAUL E. CROARKIN, DO, MS
Associate Professor of Psychiatry and Psychology, Division Chair, Child and Adolescent Psychiatry, Mayo Clinic College of Medicine & Science, Rochester, Minnesota, USA

ALLYSON WITTERS CUNDIFF, MD
Assistant Professor of Clinical Psychiatry and Behavioral Sciences, Division of Child and Adolescent Psychiatry, Vanderbilt University Medical Center, Nashville, Tennessee, USA

DIRK M. DHOSSCHE, MD, PhD
Professor, Department of Psychiatry, University of Mississippi Medical Center, Jackson, Mississippi, USA

DENIZ DORUK CAMSARI, MD
Resident in Psychiatry, Department of Psychiatry and Psychology, Division of Child and Adolescent Psychiatry, Mayo Clinic, Rochester, Minnesota, USA

ANDREW D. FRANKLIN, MD, MBA
Department of Anesthesiology, Division of Pediatric Anesthesiology, Vanderbilt University Medical Center, Nashville, Tennessee, USA

BRADLEY FREEMAN, MD
Associate Professor of Clinical Psychiatry, Department of Psychiatry and Behavioral Sciences, Vanderbilt University Medical Center, Nashville, Tennessee, USA

CATHERINE FUCHS, MD, DFAACAP
Professor of Psychiatry and Behavioral Sciences and Pediatrics, Division of Child and Adolescent Psychiatry, Vanderbilt University Medical Center, Nashville, Tennessee, USA

PAUL A. FUCHS, MD, MPH
Resident Physician, Department of Psychiatry and Behavioral Sciences, Vanderbilt University Medical Center, Nashville, Tennessee, USA

DANIEL L. KENNEY-JUNG, MD
Assistant Professor, Department of Neurology, University of Minnesota, Minneapolis, Minnesota, USA

JONATHAN C. LEE, MD, MSc
Research Fellow, Temerty Centre for Therapeutic Brain Intervention, Centre for Addiction and Mental Health, Department of Psychiatry, Faculty of Medicine, University of Toronto, Toronto, Ontario, Canada

CHARLES P. LEWIS, MD
Instructor in Psychiatry, Department of Psychiatry and Psychology, Division of Child and Adolescent Psychiatry, Mayo Clinic, Rochester, Minnesota, USA

FRANK P. MacMASTER, PhD
Associate Professor of Pediatrics and Psychiatry, Scientific Director, Strategic Clinical Network for Addictions and Mental Health, University of Calgary, Alberta Children's Hospital, Calgary, Alberta, Canada

CHRISTOPHER TODD MALEY, MD
Assistant Professor of Clinical Psychiatry, Department of Psychiatry and Behavioral Sciences, Vanderbilt University Medical Center, Vanderbilt Psychiatric Hospital, Nashville, Tennessee, USA

TODD E. PETERS, MD, FAPA
Medical Director, Child and Adolescent Services, Chief Medical Information Officer (CMIO), Sheppard Pratt Health System, Sheppard Pratt Physicians PA Clinical Operations Liaison, Baltimore, Maryland

ELIZABETH K.B. SHULTZ, DO
Assistant Professor of Clinical Psychiatry, Department of Psychiatry and Behavioral Sciences, Vanderbilt University Medical Center, Vanderbilt Psychiatric Hospital, Nashville, Tennessee, USA

JENNA H. SOBEY, MD
Department of Anesthesiology, Division of Pediatric Anesthesiology, Vanderbilt University Medical Center, Nashville, Tennessee, USA

ERIC T. STICKLES, MD
Department of Anesthesiology and Perioperative Medicine, Nemours/Alfred I. DuPont Hospital for Children, Wilmington, Delaware, USA

YASAS CHANDRA TANGUTURI, MBBS, MPH
Assistant Professor of Clinical Psychiatry and Behavioral Sciences, Division of Child and Adolescent Psychiatry, Vanderbilt University Medical Center, Nashville, Tennessee, USA

NISHA WITHANE, MD
Child Psychiatry Fellow, Department of Psychiatry, Institute of Living, Hartford Hospital, Hartford, Connecticut, USA

Contents

> The decision-making process of prescribing electroconvulsive treatment (ECT) to minors often extends outside of medicine. The legal arena is commonly involved in many jurisdictions, and some states have legislation governing the administration of this treatment in addition to hospital policies and regulations. Treatment failures, additional opinions, explicit consent, and legal tribunals are sometimes needed to deliver ECT to a minor in need. This article describes a process to which a provider can refer in navigating this confusing, and sometimes alien, pathway to provide ECT to his or her patient. Individual state statutes pertaining to ECT are provided.

> Proper planning and communication between psychiatry and anesthesiology teams is vital to conferring the greatest therapeutic benefit to children presenting for electroconvulsive therapy while minimizing risk. Anesthesia for the child undergoing electroconvulsive therapy should ideally provide deep hypnosis, ensure muscle relaxation to reduce injury, have minimal effect on seizure dynamics, and allow for rapid recovery to baseline neurologic and cardiopulmonary status. Unique factors for pediatric electroconvulsive therapy include the potential need for preoperative anxiolytic and inhalational induction of anesthesia, which must be weighed against the detrimental effects of anesthetic agents on the evoked seizure quality required for a successful treatment.

> Adolescent depression is a substantial global public health problem that contributes to academic failure, occupational impairment, deficits in social functioning, substance use disorders, teen pregnancy, and completed suicide. Existing treatment options often have suboptimal results and uncertain safety profiles. Transcranial magnetic stimulation may be a promising, brain-based intervention for adolescents with depression. Existing work has methodological weaknesses, and larger, neurodevelopmentally informed studies are urgently needed. Treatment with transcranial magnetic stimulation may modulate cortical GABAergic and glutamatergic imbalances. Future study will inform dosing approaches for TMS based on GABAergic and glutamatergic biomarkers.

Transcranial magnetic stimulation (TMS) is a treatment approved by the Food and Drug Administration for major depressive disorder (MDD). TMS is a neuromodulation technique that works by creating a focal magnetic field that induces a small electric current. Compared with other neuromodulation techniques, TMS is a noninvasive treatment modality that is generally well-tolerated. Because of the success of TMS in treating depression, there has been interest in applications for other neuropsychiatric diseases. The purpose of this article was to review potential uses for TMS for children and adolescents in conditions other than MDD.

Transcranial direct current stimulation (tDCS) involves the application of weak electric current to the scalp. tDCS may influence brain functioning through effects on cortical excitability, neural plasticity, and learning. Evidence in adults suggests promising therapeutic applications for depression, and the adverse effect profile is generally mild. Early research indicates complex interactions between tDCS and concurrent cognitive and motor tasks. Further investigation is warranted to understand how tDCS impacts processes relevant to psychiatric conditions.

Research involving transcranial direct current stimulation (tDCS) in child and adolescent psychiatry is limited. Early, short-term studies have found tDCS to be safe and well-tolerated in youth with neurodevelopmental disorders (attention-deficit hyperactivity disorder, autism, learning disorders). Preliminary data suggest potential utility in symptom reduction and improving cognitive function. Further careful research considering implications for the developing brain is necessary.

Despite the majority of patients with anti-N-methyl D-aspartate receptor (NMDAR) antibody encephalitis presenting with catatonic symptoms, the literature has not focused on well-known treatments for catatonia, such as electroconvulsive therapy (ECT). The authors review the literature identifying case reports that document the effective use of ECT for anti-NMDAR encephalitis. They also identify gaps in the literature regarding use and documentation of ECT and review possible mechanisms of action for ECT. The authors propose identifying catatonia as a syndrome with multiple potential causes (including anti-NMDAR encephalitis) and suggest a standardized treatment approach using evidence-based catatonia treatments such as ECT and benzodiazepines.

CHILD AND ADOLESCENT PSYCHIATRIC CLINICS

ISSUE OF RELATED INTEREST

Psychiatric Clinics of North America, September 2018 (Vol. 41, No. 3)
Neuromodulation
Scott T. Aaronson and Noah S. Philip, *Editors*
Available at: http://www.psych.theclinics.com/

AACAP Members: Please go to www.jaacap.org for information on access to the Child and Adolescent Psychiatric Clinics. *Resident* Members of AACAP: Special access information is available at www.childpsych.theclinics.com.

THE CLINICS ARE AVAILABLE ONLINE!
Access your subscription at:
www.theclinics.com

Preface

Neuromodulation: Past, Present, and Future

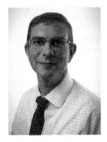 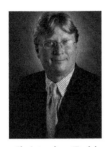 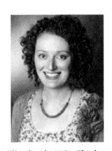 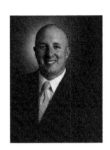

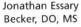

| Jonathan Essary Becker, DO, MS | Christopher Todd Maley, MD | Elizabeth K.B. Shultz, DO | Todd E. Peters, MD, FAPA |

Editors

Neuromodulation represents the oldest biological-based treatment for psychiatric illness with the development of electroconvulsive therapy (ECT) in 1938. To this day, ECT remains the most effective treatment for several psychiatric illnesses, including mania, depression, and catatonia. In addition to high remission rates, several recent studies have highlighted additional benefits of ECT, including decreased length of time in an acute episode, decreased hospital readmission, and overall cost benefit for using ECT as a second-line treatment. Despite the benefits of ECT, it is often still not considered until later in the course of treatment for many people because of the burden of repeated general anesthesia, cognitive side effects, and some lingering stigma. As a result, interest has grown in other forms of neuromodulation to explore different treatment modalities that can offer similar benefit with better tolerability. These treatments include vagal nerve stimulation, deep brain stimulation, transcranial magnetic stimulation (TMS), and direct current stimulation (DCS). Each modality provides advantages and disadvantages in the treatment of psychiatric illness.

While ECT is used less frequently in children and adolescents, it remains an important treatment in pediatric patients with severe illness, such as high suicide risk with depression, affective psychotic illnesses, and catatonia. There is also increasing interest in the use of ECT for management of aggressive and self-injurious behavior in autism spectrum disorder. In our practice, we have seen significant benefits in quality of life for both the patient and the families of these patients with significant behavioral dysregulation in autism.

With children and adolescents, patients and families may raise concern about the risks of adverse reactions to medications. This concern is highlighted by the black box warning for antidepressants in this population. TMS and DCS offer distinct

Child Adolesc Psychiatric Clin N Am 28 (2019) xi–xii
https://doi.org/10.1016/j.chc.2018.08.003
1056-4993/19/© 2018 Published by Elsevier Inc.

advantages in their safety profiles. Those wishing to avoid medications may be more open to a noninvasive neuromodulation technique with proven efficacy.

Neuromodulation remains a burgeoning field with much room for growth. Further research is needed to more definitively determine which conditions benefit from which type of therapy. Of additional importance is determining which brain regions to target with therapy as well as standardizing evidence-based treatment protocols. We believe neuromodulation has the potential to provide relief to the many patients struggling with refractory and difficult-to-treat psychiatric illnesses while minimizing long-term side effects.

Jonathan Essary Becker, DO, MS
Vanderbilt University Medical School
Department of Psychiatry and
Behavioral Sciences
1601 23rd Avenue South
Nashville, TN 37212, USA

Christopher Todd Maley, MD
Vanderbilt University Medical Center
Department of Psychiatry and
Behavioral Sciences
1601 23rd Avenue South
Nashville, TN 37212, USA

Elizabeth K.B. Shultz, DO
Vanderbilt University Medical Center
Department of Psychiatry and
Behavioral Sciences
1601 23rd Avenue South
Nashville, TN 37212, USA

Todd E. Peters, MD, FAPA
Child and Adolescent Services
Sheppard Pratt Health System
6501 North Charles Street
Baltimore, MD 21204, USA

E-mail addresses:
jonathan.e.becker@vumc.org (J.E. Becker)
christopher.maley@vumc.org (C.T. Maley)
elizabeth.shultz@vumc.org (E.K.B. Shultz)
tpeters@sheppardpratt.org (T.E. Peters)

Pathway to Electroconvulsive Treatment for Minors

Bradley Freeman, MD

KEYWORDS

- Electroconvulsive therapy • Process • Regulation • Legislation

KEY POINTS

- The pathway to electroconvulsive treatment (ECT) delivery to minors can involve multiple health care providers, the family, attorneys, judges, and committees.
- The pathway to ECT delivery is depends on the jurisdiction in which the patient is being treated.
- In many jurisdictions, ECT administration requires legal approval and adherence to local regulations and facility policy.
- There is no consistent oversight or regulation for the delivery of ECT to minors in the United States.

INTRODUCTION

Electroconvulsive therapy (ECT) remains one of the most regulated treatments in medicine.[1] Despite the work of national medical organizations, the process to undergo ECT can differ substantially from one state to another. The American Psychiatric Association (APA) has published guidelines on the treatment of moderate to severe major depressive disorder in which ECT is a recommended intervention after pharmacotherapy has failed.[2] The organization also asserts ECT as the treatment of choice for medication-resistant episodes of acute mania in individuals with bipolar disorder.[3] More specific to minors, the American Academy of Child and Adolescent Psychiatry (AACAP) has suggested ECT be considered in adolescents suffering from treatment-resistant depression or those with a severe, psychotic depression.[4] AACAP's 2007 publication also noted that the research supporting ECT in the child and adolescent population has "not been well studied." A more recent publication by Puffer and colleagues[5] examined the outcomes of 51 adolescents who received ECT and ultimately suggested ECT is a safe and effective intervention for treatment resistant youth.

Still, many child and adolescent psychiatrists have little knowledge, training, or experience in ECT. An attitudes survey of over 600 child and adolescent psychiatrists from 2001 showed that 53% of providers had minimal knowledge about ECT use in

Disclosure: The author has nothing to disclose.
Department of Psychiatry and Behavioral Sciences, Vanderbilt University Medical Center, 1601 23rd Avenue South, Suite 3023, Nashville, TN 37212, USA
E-mail address: bradley.w.freeman@vanderbilt.edu

minors; 75% lacked the confidence/skill to provide a second consultant opinion, and 52% believed ECT was unsafe in prepubertal children. Additionally, 26% thought it was dangerous in adolescents.[6] A practice parameter for ECT with adolescents was published by AACAP in 2004.[7] This work intended to guide providers in the decision-making process for utilizing ECT in adolescents and to describe the administration of ECT, potential adverse effects, and to address the legal and ethical issues of the intervention. Although there are misperceptions, confusion, and strong opponents to ECT, it is a safe and beneficial procedure with a high response rate.[8]

There are few areas in medicine in which state legislatures have been concerned. State statutes rightfully describe the liberty an individual has with regard to making their own decisions, including health care decisions. Some states, however, have specific laws governing the application of ECT of which providers in those jurisdictions must be aware. California and Alaska are guided by case law, whereas other states lack mention of ECT in their statues altogether.[9,10] California mandates patients be informed "...that there is a difference of opinion within the medical profession" regarding the utility of ECT (Aden v Younger, 1976). States do not uniformly require a specific numbers of opinions regarding the necessity of ECT for a particular patient.

The recommendations set out by the medical community are not rigidly implemented across the United States. This article attempts to help providers by offering a basic model of decision making for administration of ECT in youth. The article describes aspects of interest to providers and patients. Still, legislation and regulatory bodies are dynamic in nature. Providers should be aware of current regulations in their jurisdiction and policies at their facility.

MATERIALS AND METHODS

Published literature was reviewed with regard to legal stipulations surrounding the administration of ECT in minors. The PubMed database was queried with the various combinations of search terms including "electroconvulsive therapy," "ECT," "adolescent," "child," "regulation," and "standard." The most recent practice parameters from the APA and AACAP were reviewed, and individual state legislatures were searched using the terms "electroconvulsive," "ECT," "shock therapy," and "electroshock" from March 2018 to May 2018. The information was coalesced into a flowchart that best represents a general decision making process for the clinical and legal application of ECT to a minor. The flowchart may not be applicable to specific jurisdictions because of either a difference or change in its regulations and policies (**Fig. 1**).

RESULTS

Table 1, developed by Livingston and colleagues,[11] describes legislation surrounding consent for ECT. For the purposes of this article, minors generally fall under those individuals without decision-making capacity. There are, however, areas of the country that allow certain minors to make medical decisions. **Table 2** presents additional restrictions for the administration of ECT. Twenty-nine states including Alabama,[12] Alaska,[13] Arizona,[14] Arkansas,[15] Connecticut,[16] District of Columbia,[17] Hawaii,[18] Indiana,[19] Iowa,[20] Maine,[21] Maryland,[22] Minnesota,[23] Montana,[24] Nebraska,[25] Nevada,[26] New Hampshire,[27] New Jersey,[28] New Mexico,[29] North Carolina,[30] North Dakota,[31] Oklahoma,[32] Oregon,[33] Pennsylvania,[34] Rhode Island,[35] South Carolina,[36] Vermont,[37] Washington,[38] West Virginia,[39] Wisconsin,[40] and Wyoming[41] have no age restrictions in their legislation regarding the administration of ECT. Other states specify either a particular age limit or none at all. In states with age restrictions, they differ in their requirements surrounding the pre-ECT evaluation. The process

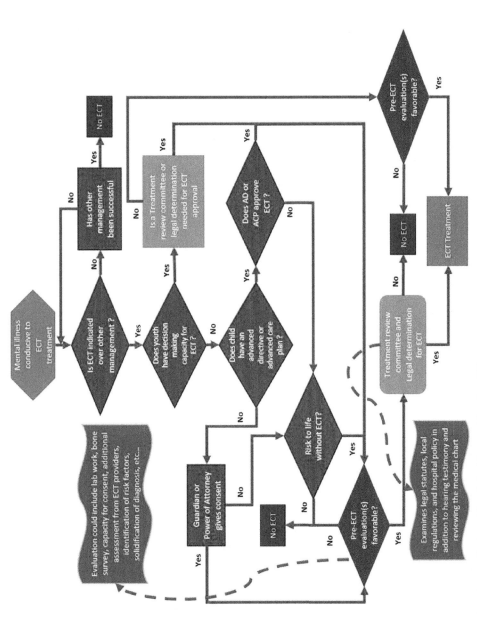

Fig. 1. Navigating the medical and legal decision making for ECT.

Table 1
Informed consent for electroconvulsive treatment by US state

State	Specific Consent Form Required	Written Consent Explicitly Required for Electroconvulsive Treatment Required	Patient Without Decision-Making Capacity
Alabama[44]			
Alaska[45]	−	+	Must have a court order unless noted in an advanced directive or has authorized a surrogate to consent
Arizona[46]			
Arkansas[47]	−	−	ECT may be given only after 72 h of hospitalization if circuit court is presented with clear and convincing proof that treatment is necessary
California[48,49]	+	+	Guardian, responsible relative, or conservator may consent.
Colorado[50]	+	+	
Connecticut[51]	−	+	If no less intrusive beneficial treatment, the probate court may order ECT to be done within 45 d.
District of Columbia[52]	−	+	Court order or legal guardian with explicit directive for ECT required.
Delaware[53]	−	+	
Florida[54]	−	+	Must have informed consent from guardian of adjudicated incapacitated patient if not due to substance abuse or from guardian advocate of patient if given expressed court authority to consent. Surrogate or proxy may not consent.
Georgia[a,55]	−	+	Advanced mental health care directive may provide consent.
Hawaii[56]	−	+	Advanced mental health care directive allows patient to have power of attorney consent.
Idaho[57]	−	−	Advanced mental health care directive includes preference on ECT with ability to assign an agent to consent.
Illinois[58]	−	+	Only a guardian may consent. If patient refuses treatment, it may be given if no less restrictive alternative exists but may be administered not in excess of 72 h without a court hearing approving further treatment.
Indiana[59]	−	+	Appointed individual may consent.
Iowa[60]	−	+	May be given only if treatment is necessary to protect health or safety of the individual or is ordered by the court.
Kansas[61]	−	+	

State	–	+	Notes
Kentucky[62]	–	+	Advanced mental health care directive includes ability to consent.
Louisiana[63]	–	+	Director of treatment facility can apply for court to determine competence. Or, if the director consults 2 physicians who agree the condition of a patient who is incapable of informed consent is life threatening, ECT may be administered.
Maine[64]	–	+	Consent from a court of competent jurisdiction, a guardian, or other legal decision maker is required. Hearing officer cannot order ECT.
Maryland[65]			
Massachusetts[66]	–	+	Review and approval by court of competent jurisdiction or consent of legally authorized representative are required.
Michigan[67]	–	+	May obtain consent from guardian/designated representative. If guardian consents, shall not be initiated until 2 psychiatrists have examined and documented concurrent with decision to administer. If representative cannot be located, probate court may consent.
Minnesota[68]	–	+	Advanced directive may provide consent except in emergencies. No guardian may give consent unless treatment is court ordered.
Mississippi[69]	–	+	Informed consent from patient's family or legal guardian required.
Missouri[70]	–	+	Legal guardian must obtain a court order for treatment. If approved, court may order number of treatments in a specified time period.
Montana[71]	–	+	Advanced mental health care directive may provide consent.
Nebraska[72]			
Nevada[73]			
New Hampshire[74]	–		Guardian may not give consent unless first approved by probate court order.
New Jersey[75]	–	+	Court may hold a hearing to determine necessity.
New Mexico[76]			
New York[77]	–	+	
North Carolina[78]	–	+	Consent of legally responsible person, health care agent named pursuant to a valid health care power of attorney, or client's consent expressed in a valid advance instruction required.
North Dakota[79]	–	+ May give oral consent with 2 witnesses not part of treatment team	Informed written consent of guardian required.

(continued on next page)

Table 1
(continued)

State	Specific Consent Form Required	Written Consent Explicitly for Electroconvulsive Treatment Required	Patient Without Decision-Making Capacity
Ohio[80]	−	+	Guardian may consent. Chief clinical officer may recommend administration if there is no guardian. Without durable power of attorney, decision goes to court.
Oklahoma[81]	−	+	Advanced mental health care directive may provide consent.
Oregon[82]	−	−	Health care representative may not give consent. Mental health declaration may provide consent.
Pennsylvania[83]	−	+	Preferences and designated agents may be detailed in declaration of mental health form.
Rhode Island[84]			
South Carolina[85]	−	+	If attending physician or physician on call decides ECT is necessary, guardian or persons in order of priority may consent.
South Dakota[86]	−	+	In emergency, if 2 physicians determine necessity, ECT may be continued up to 10 d and can be extended with petition to court for mental illness who may authorize treatment. Necessity reviewed every 30 d with court able to approve up to 1 y.
Tennessee[87]	−	+	Preferences may be detailed by a mental health declaration.
Texas[88]	+	+	Legal guardian may consent.
Utah[89]	−	+	Patient's family or legal guardian may consent.
Vermont[90]	+	+	
Virginia[91]	−	+	
Washington[92]	−	+	Involuntarily committed patient's lack of consent may be overridden by a hearing.
West Virginia[93]			
Wisconsin[94]	−	+	Guardian may consent.
Wyoming[95]	−	−	Upon order of court, guardian may consent.

a Nothing in state law currently, but under review this year in the state House of Representatives and Senate.

From Livingston R, Wu C, Mu K, et al. Regulation of electroconvulsive therapy: a systematic review of US State laws. J ECT 2018;34(1): 61–2; with permission.

Table 2
Regulatory requirements for electroconvulsive treatment practice by US state

State	Age Restrictions	Qualified Professional	Reporting Guidelines	Other
Alabama[44]		Psychologists and marriage/family therapists may not administer.		
Alaska[45]				
Arizona[46]				
Arkansas[47]				
California[48,49]	<12 y old—no ECT 12–16 y—only if emergency situation and ECT deemed lifesaving, 3 child psychiatrists appointed by the local mental health director agree, and thoroughly documented and reported to the director of Health Care Services Voluntary patients aged 16–17 y old—may grant/withhold consent to the same extent as adult voluntary patient	May only be performed by a physician licensed in California. Psychologists may not administer.	Quarterly	Details appointed members of ECT review committee and their function Persons with developmental disabilities admitted or committed to hospital may refuse No more than 15 treatments within 30-d period or >30 treatments within 1-y period To exceed–prior approval must be obtained from review committee of facility or county—maximum number of additional treatments shall be specified
Colorado[50]	<16 y old—no ECT 16–18 y—approval of 2 psychiatrists and a parent/guardian must recommend/consent >18 y old–2 psychiatrists determine that ECT is most preferred form of treatment		Semiannually	

(continued on next page)

Table 2
(continued)

State	Age Restrictions	Qualified Professional	Reporting Guidelines	Other
Connecticut[51]				$250 to file application with probate court to authorize ECT
District of Columbia[52]				
Delaware[53]	<18 y old—requires legal guardian consent	Psychologists may not administer		
Florida[54]	<18 y old—requires legal guardian consent	Clinical social workers, marriage/family therapists, mental health counsellors may not administer		Record must be reviewed by one other physician not involved in patient's care, who documents agreement with treatment
Georgia[a,55]	<16 y old—no ECT	May only be administered by ECT licensed physician	Annually	
Hawaii[56]				
Idaho[57]	<18 y old—no ECT except by court order			
Illinois[58]	<18 y old—requires parent/legal guardian consent and must be approved by court—2 licensed psychiatrists must evaluate and agree with need for ECT	May only be performed by a physician or nurse with physician supervision	Quarterly	Department shall conduct annual trainings for all physicians and registered nurses working in state-operated mental health facilities on appropriate use of ECT
Indiana[59]				
Iowa[60]				
Kansas[61]	<18 y old—requires legal guardian consent with court approval to consent for ECT			
Kentucky[62]	Court cannot order consent to treatment in minors			

State	Provision	Frequency	Additional
Louisiana[63]	No minors confined by emergency certificate/commitment/court order can receive ECT without written consent of a court after a hearing. However, if director of treatment facility and 2 physicians determine that it is so critical that it may be life-threatening without, emergency measures may be performed without consent		
Maine[64]			
Maryland[65]			
Massachusetts[66]	<16 y old–no ECT unless commissioner or designee concurs	Monthly	Facility shall establish written plan for administration of ECT in compliance with standards
Michigan[67]	<18 y old–parent who has legal and physical custody must give consent. Minor or advocate designated by minor may object to ECT. ECT shall not be initiated before court hearing on minor's or advocate's objection. If parent or guardian of a minor consents to ECT, shall not be initiated until 2 child and adolescent psychiatrists, neither of whom may be the treating psychiatrist, document concurrence to administer		
Minnesota[68]			
Mississippi[69]	Shall not be administered to children or adolescents unless 2 qualified child and adolescent psychiatrists who are not affiliated with treating program concur with decision to administer		Use of ECT and other forms of convulsive therapy requires special justification

(continued on next page)

Table 2
(continued)

State	Age Restrictions	Qualified Professional	Reporting Guidelines	Other
Missouri[70]	Parents of minors are required to obtain court order.			Persons solely diagnosed as intellectually disabled are not subject to ECT
Montana[71]		Psychologist may not administer		Electric shock devices are considered research techniques for those with developmental disabilities and may only be used in extraordinary circumstances to prevent self-mutilation leading to repeated and possibly permanent physical damage only if alternative techniques have failed
Nebraska[72]		Social worker may not administer		
Nevada[73]		Clinical professional counselor may not administer		
New Hampshire[74]				
New Jersey[75]				
New Mexico[76]				
New York[77]	<16 y old–no ECT >65 y old–2 physicians must state necessity	May only be administered by a physician	Quarterly reports to state, compiled annually to governor	Equipment registration/fee required

State			
North Carolina[78]			
North Dakota[79]			Treating those with developmental disabilities requires written consent (if minor, requires parent/guardian written informed consent)
Ohio[80]	<18 y old–no ECT		Identifies first-line uses Details required medical workup
Oklahoma[81]		Psychologist may not administer	
Oregon[82]			
Pennsylvania[83]			
Rhode Island[84]			
South Carolina[85]			
South Dakota[86]	>16 y old–may refuse whether involuntarily committed or admitted by parent If treatment is prescribed by treating psychiatrist and agreed upon by another physician, treatment may be administered with informed consent of minor's parent, guardian, or other legal custodian pending judicial determination	May only be administered by a physician	

(continued on next page)

Table 2
(continued)

State	Age Restrictions	Qualified Professional	Reporting Guidelines	Other
Tennessee[87]	May treat children with mania or severe depression if all other accepted therapies have been exhausted or necessary to save child's life because of potential suicide or to prevent irreparable injury Multidisciplinary review of at least 5 persons (at least 1 independent of service provider) approves ECT and American Board of Psychiatry and Neurology (ABPN)-certified child and adolescent psychiatrist approves >14 y old–requires second ABPN psychiatrist approval, child does not object after being informed, and at least 1 parent or legal guardian consents		Annually	
Texas[88]	<16 y old–no ECT >16 y old can be treated if guardian consents >65 y old–2 physicians must concur treatment is medically necessary	May only be administered by a physician	Quarterly reports to state, compiled annually to governor	Details required medical work-up No more than 15 treatments within an 8-wk period or 24 in a 12-mo period without the concurrence of a qualified psychiatrist not involved in the patient's care ECT equipment must be registered annually ($50)

State		Commissioner collects statistical data	Commissioner of Mental Health oversees and monitors all facilities administering ECT
Utah[89]	Regardless of whether child/guardian agrees/disagrees with proposed ECT, due process procedure shall be conducted prior to administration		
Vermont[90]		Commissioner collects statistical data	Commissioner of Mental Health oversees and monitors all facilities administering ECT
Virginia[91]	<18 y old–2 qualified child psychiatrists (not directly involved in treating the child) must concur with treatment		
Washington[92]			
West Virginia[93]			
Wisconsin[94]	May only be administered under direct supervision of a physician		
Wyoming[95]			

[a] Nothing in state law currently, but under review this year in House of Representatives and Senate.

From Livingston R, Wu C, Mu K, et al. Regulation of electroconvulsive therapy: a systematic review of US State laws. J ECT 2018;34(1): 63–6; with permission.

of approving the use of ECT can be complicated, and institutions have worked to develop procedural guidelines.[42]

Fig. 1 represents a pathway the treating provider can follow regarding ECT approval for minors. The provider must first identify if ECT is indicated as a treatment intervention for the patient's mental illness. The first step involves deciding if other forms of management are preferred or indicated. If other acceptable management strategies have failed, then ECT can be discussed with the patient and guardian. Some children have decision making capacity and will be able to provide their own informed consent for the procedure. For example, the California statute indicates voluntary patients aged 16 and 17 can provide consent in the same way as a voluntary adult. Although uncommon, there are some children who have advanced directives that help guide the decision-making process.

If the child does not have an advanced directive, consent is sought from the child's guardian such as the family or power of attorney. If the guardian approves the treatment, then a legal determination is made concerning the ability to provide ECT to the patient. The legal determination is based on the jurisdictional requirements, current legislation, and hospital policies. If the provider is legally allowed to proceed, then a course of ECT can be administered. In many institutions, a treatment review committee (TRC) is also convened to discuss this intervention on a particular patient.

During the process of decision-making and ECT administration, the health care decision maker can terminate the process at any step. Additionally, pre-ECT evaluations are typically completed after the guardian has consented to the procedure but before the TRC or legal determinations have been made. There are several hard stops in the process, the most obvious being the wishes of the health care decision maker.

DISCUSSION

Prescribing ECT for minors is not a simple undertaking and requires some effort and advocacy on the part of the health care provider and/or treatment team. There has been opposition to the treatment and unnecessary stigma, which is difficult to overcome. The decision-making model described in this article is meant to offer general guidance for the providers. The process can take several days to weeks in some circumstances and active treatment can be disrupted if the patient relocates to a new jurisdiction with different rules governing the use of ECT.

Navigating the decision-making process to administer ECT is challenging for the providers and the patient and his or her family. Families originally accepting of ECT treatment have become resistant once the legal system becomes involved. The inclusion of attorneys and judges can suggest the treatment is more dangerous and serious than originally thought, resulting in an increase in anxiety and withdrawal of consent. There are few other treatments in medicine so regulated by people who are not health care providers. For instance, various pediatric surgical procedures with greater risk of harm than ECT do not require such legal oversight. Additionally, health care providers are not expected to be familiar with the legal arena. This unfamiliarity can be a deterrent to prescribing ECT for a patient.

An institutional's TRC may be involved in the decision to move forward with ECT. This committee ensures the necessity of the treatment for the patient as well as conformation with institutional and regional policy and regulations. A TRC also helps providers decide on treatment for involuntary patients. The ability for persons to consent to ECT is often questioned because of the severity of their mental illness. Persons in the throes of an acute manic episode or suffering from a catatonic depression may have difficulty forming the cognitive functions to give informed consent. The

TRC is an effective pause in the process of determining whether ECT can be provided to a patient.

As previously noted, there are several hard stops with regard to the ECT decision-making process. These include factors such as a not identifying an indication for the treatment, informed consent not being provided, lack of necessity when informed consent is not provided, failure to meet legal and facility requirements, and contraindications specific to the patient that prevent the administration of ECT (eg, unstable angina, recent stroke, or pheochromocytoma).[43]

Health care providers should continue to advocate for their patients. They must work to eliminate barriers so their patients can receive the treatment they need. With ECT, these barriers exist in areas outside of medicine that can deter some providers on moving forward. Patients are also encouraged to advocate for access to necessary treatments. Of course, additional ECT research in the juvenile population would be welcomed.

REFERENCES

1. Harris V. Electroconvulsive therapy: administrative codes, legislation, and professional recommendations. J Am Acad Psychiatry Law 2006;34:406–11.
2. American Psychiatric Association. Practice guidelines for the treatment of patients with major depressive disorder. Am J Psychiatry 2000;157(Suppl 4): 1–45.
3. American Psychiatric Association. Practice guidelines for the treatment of patients with bipolar disorder (revision). Am J Psychiatry 1994;151(Suppl 12):1–35.
4. American Academy of Child & Adolescent Psychiatry. Practice parameter for the assessment and treatment of children and adolescents with depressive disorders. J Am Acad Child Adolesc Psychiatry 2007;46(11):1503–26.
5. Puffer C, Wall C, Huxsahl J, et al. A 20 year practice review of electroconvulsive therapy for adolescents. J Child Adolesc Psychopharmacol 2016;26(7):632–6.
6. Ghaziuddin N, Kaza M, Ghazi N, et al. Electroconvulsive therapy for minors: experiences and attitudes of child psychiatrists and psychologists. J ECT 2001;17: 109–17.
7. American Academy of Child & Adolescent Psychiatry. Practice parameter for use of electroconvulsive therapy with adolescents. J Am Acad Child Adolesc Psychiatry 2004;43(12):1521–39.
8. Sachs M, Madaan V. Electroconvulsive therapy in children and adolescents: brief overview and ethical issues. AACAP Ethics Committee; 2012. Available at: https://www.aacap.org/App_Themes/AACAP/docs/member_resources/ethics/in_ workplace/Sachs_Maadan_Electroconvulsive_Therapy_in_children_and_adolescents. pdf. Accessed May 11, 2018.
9. Aden v. Younger, 129 Cal. Rptr. 535 (Cal. Ct. App. 1976).
10. Wyatt v. Hardin, 1975 U.S. Dist. LEXIS 13571 (M.D. Ala. 1975).
11. Livingston R, Wu C, Mu K, et al. Regulation of electroconvulsive therapy: a systematic review of US State laws. J ECT 2018;34:60–8.
12. Legislature from the State of Alabama. Available at: http://alisondb.legislature. state.al.us/alison/CoaSearchContent.aspx. Accessed May 10, 2018.
13. Legislature from the State of Alaska. Available at: http://www.legis.state.ak.us/ basis/folio.asp. Accessed May 10, 2018.
14. Legislature from the State of Arizona. Available at: http://www.azleg.gov. Accessed May 10, 2018.

15. Legislature from the State of Arkansas. Available at: http://www.lexisnexis.com/hottopics/arcode/Default.asp. Accessed May 10, 2018.

16. Legislature from the State of Connecticut's General Assembly. Available at: https://search.cga.state.ct.us/r/statute/. Accessed May 10, 2018.

17. Legislature from the District of Columbia Code. Available at: http://dccode.elaws.us. Accessed May 10, 2018.

18. Legislature from the State of Hawaii. Available at: http://www.capitol.hawaii.gov. Accessed May 10, 2018.

19. Legislature from the State of Indiana. Find Law: Indiana Code. Available at: http://codes.findlaw.com/in/title-16-health/in-code-sect-16-36-1-7-3.html. Accessed May 10, 2018.

20. Legislature from the State of Iowa. Available at: https://www.legis.iowa.gov/publications/search/document?fq=id:491043&pdid=701814&q=electroconvulsive #441.29.6. Accessed May 10, 2018.

21. Legislature from the State of Maine. Available at: http://www.maine.gov/dhhs/samhs/mentalhealth/rights-legal/index.html. Accessed May 10, 2018.

22. Legislature from the State of Maryland's General Assembly. Available at: http://mgaleg.maryland.gov/webmga/frmStatutes.aspx?pid=statpage&tab=subject5. Accessed May 10, 2018.

23. Legislature from the State of Minnesota. Office of the Revisor of Statutes. Available at: https://www.revisor.mn.gov/laws. Accessed May 10, 2018.

24. Legislature from the State of Minnesota. Available at: http://search.leg.mt.gov. Accessed May 10, 2018.

25. Legislature from the State of Nebraska. Available at: http://www.sos.ne.gov/rules-and-regs/regsearch/index.html. Accessed May 10, 2018.

26. Legislature from the State of Nevada. Available at: https://www.leg.state.nv.us/Site/Search/search.cfm. Accessed May 10, 2018.

27. Legislature from the State of New Hampshire. Revised Statutes Online. Available at: http://www.gencourt.state.nh.us/rsa/html/indexes/search.html. Accessed May 10, 2018.

28. Legislature from the State of New Jersey. Available at: http://lis.njleg.state.nj.us/nxt/gateway.dll?f=templates&fn=default.htm&vid=Publish:10.1048/Enu. Accessed May 10, 2018.

29. Legislature from the State of New Mexico. Available at: https://nmlegis.gov/. Accessed May 10, 2018.

30. Legislature from the State of North Carolina's General Assembly. Available at: http://www.ncga.state.nc.us/gascripts/statutes/Statutes.asp. Accessed May 10, 2018.

31. Legislature from the State of North Dakota. Available at: http://www.legis.nd.gov/search. Accessed May 10, 2018.

32. Legislature from the State of Oklahoma State. Available at: http://oklegislature.gov/. Accessed May 10, 2018.

33. Legislature from the State of Oregon State. Available at: https://www.oregonlegislature.gov/. Accessed May 10, 2018.

34. Legislature from the State of Pennsylvania. Available at: http://www.legis.state.pa.us/cfdocs/legis/li/public/. Accessed May 10, 2018.

35. Legislature from the State of Rhode Island's General Assembly. Available at: http://webserver.rilin.state.ri.us/Statutes. Accessed May 10, 2018.

36. Legislature from the State of South Carolina. Available at: http://www.scstatehouse.gov/query.php?search=FIRST&searchtext=&category=CODEOFLAWS. Accessed May 10, 2018.

37. Legislature from the State of Vermont's General Assembly. Available at: http://legislature.vermont.gov/statutes/search. Accessed May 10, 2018.

38. Legislature from the State of Washington. Available at: http://search.leg.wa.gov/. Accessed May 10, 2018.

39. Legislature from the State of West Virginia. Available at: http://www.legis.state.wv.us/WVCODE/Code.cfm. Accessed May 10, 2018.

40. Legislature from the State of Wisconsin State. Available at: http://docs.legis.wisconsin.gov. Accessed May 10, 2018.

41. Legislature from the State of Wyoming. LexisNexis Wyoming Statutes Public Access. Available at: http://www.lexisnexis.com/hottopics/wystatutes/. Accessed May 10, 2018.

42. Canberra Hospital and Health Services Clinical Procedure. Electroconvulsive therapy (ECT) – adults and children over 12 years of age. Available at: http://www.health.act.gov.au/sites/default/files//new_policy_and_plan/Electroconvulsive%20Therapy%20%28ECT%29%20-%20Adults%20and%20Children%20over%2012%20years%20of%20age.docx. Accessed May 12, 2018.

43. Zis A. Introduction to electroconvulsive therapy. Biol Psychiatry 2000;26:611–21.

44. The Alabama Legislature. Available at: http://alisondb.legislature.state.al.us/alison/CoaSearchContent.aspx. Accessed April 7, 2017.

45. The Alaska State Legislature. Available at: http://www.legis.state.ak.us/basis/folio.asp. Accessed March 29, 2017.

46. Arizona State Legislature. Available at: http://www.azleg.gov. Accessed March 29, 2017.

47. Arkansas Code. Available at: http://www.lexisnexis.com/hottopics/arcode/Default.asp. Accessed March 29, 2017.

48. California Legislative Information. Available at: http://leginfo.legislature.ca.gov/faces/codes.xhtml. Accessed March 31, 2017.

49. California Code of Regulations. Available at: https://govt.westlaw.com/calregs/index?__lrTS=20170331163747673&transitionType=Default&contextData=(sc.Default). Accessed March 31, 2017.

50. Colorado Revised Statutes. Available at: https://www.lexisnexis.com/hottopics/colorado/. Accessed April 10, 2017.

51. Connecticut General Assembly. Available at: https://www.cga.ct.gov. Accessed April 10, 2017.

52. District of Columbia Code. Available at: http://dccode.elaws.us. Accessed April 10, 2017.

53. The Delaware Code Online. Available at: http://delcode.delaware.gov. Accessed April 26, 2017.

54. The Florida Statutes. Available at: http://www.leg.state.fl.us/Statutes. Accessed April 27, 2017.

55. Georgia General Assembly. Available at: http://www.legis.ga.gov/en-US/default.aspx. Accessed April 27, 2017.

56. Hawaii State Legislature. Available at: http://www.capitol.hawaii.gov. Accessed May 8, 2017.

57. Idaho State Legislature. Available at: https://legislature.idaho.gov. Accessed May, 10 2017.

58. Illinois General Assembly. Available at: http://www.ilga.gov/legislation/ilcs/ilcs5.asp?ActID=1496&ChapterID=34. Accessed April 25, 2017.

59. Find Law: Indiana Code. Available at: http://codes.findlaw.com/in/title-16-health/in-code-sect-16-36-1-7-3.html. Accessed April 25, 2017.

60. The Iowa Legislature. Available at: https://www.legis.iowa.gov/publications/search/document?fq=id:491043&pdid=701814&q=electroconvulsive#441.29.6. Accessed April 25, 2017.

61. Kansas Legislative Sessions. Available at: http://www.kslegislature.org/li/b2017_18/statute/. Accessed April 25, 2017.

62. Kentucky Legislature. Available at: http://www.lrc.ky.gov/statutes/search.aspx. Accessed April 25, 2017.

63. Louisiana State Legislature. Available at: http://legis.la.gov/Legis/LawSearch.aspx. Accessed April 25, 2017.

64. State of Maine. Available at: http://www.maine.gov/dhhs/samhs/mentalhealth/rights-legal/index.html. Accessed April 25, 2017.

65. General Assembly of Maryland. Available at: http://mgaleg.maryland.gov/webmga/frmStatutes.aspx?pid=statpage&tab=subject5. Accessed April 25, 2017.

66. The official Web site of the Commonwealth of Massachusetts. Available at: http://www.mass.gov/portal/government/legislative/. Accessed April 27, 2017.

67. Michigan Legislature. Available at: http://www.legislature.mi.gov/(S(11gqmyeofsedx5gr4rqp0vwf))/mileg.aspx?page=MCLBasicSearch. Accessed April 27, 2017.

68. Minnesota Legislature—Office of the Revisor of Statutes. Available at: https://www.revisor.mn.gov/search/?stat=1&laws=1&rule=1. Accessed April 27, 2017.

69. Mississippi State Department of Health. Available at: http://msdh.ms.gov/msdhsite/_static/4,1422,207.html. Accessed April 27, 2017.

70. Missouri General Assembly. Available at: http://www.moga.mo.gov/htmlpages2/statuteconstitutionsearch.aspx. Accessed April 27, 2017.

71. Search the Montana Legislature Web site. Available at: https://leg.mt.gov/bills/mca/index.html. Accessed April 25, 2017.

72. Official Nebraska government Web site. Available at: http://www.sos.ne.gov/rules-and-regs/regsearch/index.html. Accessed April 25, 2017.

73. Nevada Legislature. Available at: https://www.leg.state.nv.us/Site/Search/search.cfm. Accessed April 25, 2017.

74. State of New Hampshire revised statutes online. Available at: http://www.gencourt.state.nh.us/rsa/html/indexes/search.html. Accessed April 25, 2017.

75. New Jersey Legislature. Available at: http://lis.njleg.state.nj.us/nxt/gateway.dll?f=templates&fn=default.htm&vid=Publish:10.1048/Enu. Accessed April 25, 2017.

76. New Mexico Legislature. Available at: https://nmlegis.gov/. Accessed April 25, 2017.

77. New York State Legislature. Available at: http://public.leginfo.state.ny.us/lawssrch.cgi?NVLWO. Accessed April 25, 2017.

78. North Carolina General Assembly. Available at: http://www.ncga.state.nc.us/gascripts/statutes/Statutes.asp. Accessed April 25, 2017.

79. North Dakota Legislative Branch. Available at: http://www.legis.nd.gov/search. Accessed April 25, 2017.

80. LAWriter Ohio Laws and Rules. Available at: http://codes.ohio.gov/. Accessed April 25, 2017.

81. Oklahoma State Legislature. Available at: http://oklegislature.gov/. Accessed May 9, 2017.

82. Oregon State Legislature. Available at: https://www.oregonlegislature.gov/. Accessed May 9, 2017.

83. Unofficial Purdon's Pennsylvania statutes From Westlaw. Available at: https://govt.westlaw.com/pac/Search/Index. Accessed May 10, 2017.

84. State of Rhode Island General Assembly. Available at: http://webserver.rilin.state.ri.us/Statutes. Accessed May 9, 2017.

85. South Carolina Legislature. Available at: http://www.scstatehouse.gov/query. php?search=FIRST&searchtext=&category=CODEOFLAWS. Accessed May 9, 2017.
86. South Dakota Legislature Legislative Research Council. Available at: http:// sdlegislature.gov/statutes/Codified_Laws/TextSearch.aspx. Accessed May 9, 2017.
87. LexisNexis Tennessee code unannotated—free public access. Available at: http://www.lexisnexis.com/hottopics/tncode/. Accessed May 9, 2017.
88. Texas Constitution and statutes. Available at: http://www.statutes.legis.state.tx.us/ Search.aspx. Accessed May 9, 2017.
89. Utah State Legislature. Available at: https://le.utah.gov/solrsearch.jsp. Accessed May 9, 2017.
90. Vermont General Assembly. Available at: http://legislature.vermont.gov/statutes/ search. Accessed May 8, 2017.
91. Virginia's Legislative information system. Available at: http://law.lis.virginia.gov/ vacode. Accessed May 8, 2017.
92. Washington State Legislature. Available at: http://search.leg.wa.gov/search. aspx#document&searchQuery=&searchBase=RCW&exec=false. Accessed May 8, 2017.
93. West Virginia Legislature. Available at: http://www.legis.state.wv.us/WVCODE/ Code.cfm. Accessed May 8, 2017.
94. Wisconsin State Legislature. Available at: http://docs.legis.wisconsin.gov. Accessed May 8, 2017.
95. LexisNexioatutes annotated—free public access. Available at: http://www. lexisnexis.com/hottopics/wystatutes/. Accessed May 8, 2017.

Pediatric Electroconvulsive Therapy

An Anesthesiologist's Perspective

Andrew D. Franklin, MD, MBA[a],*, Jenna H. Sobey, MD[a],
Eric T. Stickles, MD[b]

KEYWORDS

- Electroconvulsive therapy • Pediatrics • Pediatric psychiatry • Status epilepticus
- Intravenous anesthesia • Methohexital

KEY POINTS

- Ongoing collaboration and open lines of communication between multidisciplinary teams is key to the development of a successful pediatric electroconvulsive therapy program.
- Anesthesia planning for pediatric electroconvulsive therapy is divided into preprocedural, intraprocedural, and postprocedural phases.
- Anesthesia for pediatric electroconvulsive therapy should provide deep hypnosis and muscle relaxation, impart minimal effects on seizure dynamics, and allow for rapid recovery to baseline physiologic status.

INTRODUCTION

Electroconvulsive therapy (ECT) is indicated for a variety of childhood psychiatric diseases. General anesthesia is typically administered for this brief but very stimulating procedure. There are several reports on the anesthetic management of adults undergoing ECT,[1] but robust reviews addressing the unique pediatric implications and management strategies is lacking in the medical literature. The anesthesiologist takes into consideration preprocedural, procedural, and postprocedural factors when preparing to care for a child presenting for ECT.

Disclosure Statement: All authors of this article declare no commercial or financial conflicts of interest. No funding or extra-departmental support was required for the preparation of this article. The authors have no conflict of interest. No ethical approval or funding was required for the writing of this article.

[a] Department of Anesthesiology, Division of Pediatric Anesthesiology, Vanderbilt University Medical Center, 2200 Children's Way, Suite 3115, Nashville, TN 37232, USA; [b] Department of Anesthesiology and Perioperative Medicine, Nemours/Alfred I. DuPont Hospital for Children, 1600 Rockland Road, Wilmington, DE 19803, USA
* Corresponding author.
E-mail address: andrew.franklin@vanderbilt.edu

Child Adolesc Psychiatric Clin N Am 28 (2019) 21–32
https://doi.org/10.1016/j.chc.2018.07.002
1056-4993/19/© 2018 Elsevier Inc. All rights reserved.

Preprocedural Considerations

Planning ECT for children should resemble periprocedural planning for any pediatric ambulatory surgical procedure. Fasting guidelines should be closely followed to reduce the risk of pulmonary aspiration, but clear liquids should be encouraged up to 2 hours before the procedure. The anesthesiologist should perform a preprocedural history and physical examination immediately before the procedure and consent for the anesthetic should be obtained from the parent or guardian after discussion of risks, alternatives, and benefits. Children with significant coexisting disease should be evaluated several days before the procedure to allow time for proper planning of the anesthetic as well as potential need for overnight admission to the hospital for monitoring. There are relatively few absolute contraindications for ECT from the standpoint of the psychiatrist, because ECT has been successfully applied to adult and adolescent patients with central nervous system (CNS) malignancies, hydrocephalus, and a variety of cardiopulmonary diseases. However, the anesthesiologist must carefully consider the impact anesthetic agents and the normal cardiovascular responses to ECT will have on a child's coexisting disease because he/she will be expected to treat any immediate physiologic derangements incurred during or after the procedure. A relatively new application of pediatric ECT is for salvage therapy for children in refractory status epilepticus (RSE). Although many children in RSE may be intubated and chemically sedated in the intensive care unit, the anesthesiologist may be consulted to assist, particularly if the critical care team is unfamiliar with the ECT technique and the hemodynamic manifestations that may be seen during treatment.

Many children presenting for ECT will be on at least one class of psychotropic agent that may interact with standard anesthetic agents. In general, the anesthesiologist should avoid disruption of these regularly scheduled agents given that most children presenting for ECT often critically depend on their psychotropic regimen for mood stabilization. Stimulants such as methylphenidate or dextromethorphan are occasionally used to treat children with severe depression exhibiting catatonic features and may cause resistance to agents used to induce anesthesia. Some antiepileptic agents such as phenytoin, phenobarbital, oxcarbazepine, and topiramate are potent inducers of cytochrome p-450 enzyme systems, whereas valproate is an inhibitor. These effects may affect anesthetic drug requirements and clearance. Lastly, newer atypical antipsychotics have eclipsed haloperidol due to lower risk of tardive dyskinesia in the treatment of schizophrenia, bipolar disorder, or intermittent agitation but may be associated with QTc prolongation, hypotension, anticholinergic symptoms, and prolonged sedation after anesthesia.[2] Some combative or self-injurious patients may be on scheduled or intermittent benzodiazepine agents to control symptoms, and the anesthesiologist must work closely with the psychiatrist to limit the doses of these agents before the procedure to ensure the best conditions for ECT.

Anesthesia for the child undergoing ECT should ideally provide deep hypnosis, ensure muscle relaxation to reduce injury, have minimal effect on seizure dynamics, and allow for rapid recovery to baseline neurologic and cardiopulmonary status.[3] Special attention should be given to the child's baseline neurocognitive level, airway examination, and cardiopulmonary status.

The standard physiologic monitors recommended by the American Society of Anesthesiologists (ASA) for patients receiving general anesthesia are pulse oximetry, capnography, electrocardiography, noninvasive blood pressure monitoring, and temperature monitoring. These standard ASA noninvasive monitors should be adequate for most children who do not have significant cardiopulmonary comorbidities. Bispectral index monitoring (BIS) may be considered if the anesthesiologist and psychiatrist wish to correlate anesthetic depth to the timing of the electrical stimulus, because there is some evidence to suggest that higher BIS values at seizure onset may be related to higher seizure quality.[4] Regarding airway management, appropriately sized bag-valve-mask circuits to provide positive pressure ventilation during the brief period of apnea should be available. In addition, age-/weight-appropriate airway adjuncts such as oral airways, nasal airways, laryngeal mask airways, endotracheal tubes, and laryngoscopes should be readily available to provide advanced airway support. The location of scalp electrode placement influences the portion of the child's brain that the electric current passes through, and the particular placement of electrodes with associated wires may affect the anesthesiologist's ability to properly manage the airway. Scalp electrode positioning should be discussed before induction of anesthesia. Although interpretation of the electroencephalogram (EEG) signals induction and termination of the seizure, some pediatric psychiatrists may wish to observe tonic-clonic movements of an extremity, typically the right foot, to confirm seizure activity. Electromyogram may be used by placing a right temporal electrode, which would correspond to motor movement of the right foot during the seizure. Alternatively, a blood pressure cuff on the right lower extremity may be inflated before injection of an intravenous muscle relaxant to allow the psychiatrist to observe tonic-clonic movement of the child's foot. With proper planning and execution, the entire pediatric ECT procedure can be completed within 15 minutes with subsequent transfer of the child to the postanesthesia recovery area for emergence from anesthesia. Most children may be treated and discharged on the same day, either to home or, if indicted, to a psychiatric inpatient setting. Resuscitation medications specific for pediatric patients should be nearby, preferably within an appropriately stocked pediatric resuscitation cart. Appropriate facilities and personnel to recover the child during emergence of anesthesia should be secured before the procedure, with recovery room nursing staff certified in pediatric advanced life support readily available.

The anesthesiologist makes the decision to proceed with an inhalational or intravenous induction of anesthesia for pediatric ECT based on the child's coexisting disease; level of cooperation; and effect of anesthetic technique on seizure induction, duration, and quality. Intravenous sedative-hypnotic agents have classically been given before muscle relaxation to provide brief, but potent sedation for ECT. The number of treatments required will vary considerably based on the underlying pediatric psychiatric disease and the response to initial ECT sessions. Maintenance of adequate intravenous access on inpatients scheduled for repeat treatments is important. For children scheduled for several weeks of sequential outpatient treatments, repeated awake venipuncture will likely be unnecessarily traumatic. In these situations, placement of a peripherally inserted central catheter is a reasonable consideration. Inhalational induction of general anesthesia using potent volatile anesthetic agents is useful for children with needle phobia. Because of changing pulmonary physiology, inhalational induction of general anesthesia poses greater hazard to the patient older than 12 years of age and increased risks of airway compromise during the induction phase are often seen. The degree of psychiatric illness may preclude venipuncture in the unsedated child, and inhalational induction may be the safest strategy for both the patient and the health care provider. The effects of volatile agents on the quality of the treatment are discussed later. Oral or intramuscular premedication commonly given to the pediatric patient to facilitate parental separation, anxiolysis, or sedation before venipuncture may have significant effects on the quality of the ECT (**Table 1**).

Finally, the anesthesiologist must be sensitive to the child's and family unit's need for privacy given the often negative public opinion of ECT and, unfortunately, pediatric psychiatric disease as a whole. A private preoperative holding room should be

Table 1
Anxiolytics used for pediatric electroconvulsive therapy

Agent	Suggested Dose and Route	Comments
Ketamine	0.25–0.5 mg/kg IV 5 mg/kg PO 3 mg/kg IN 5 mg/kg IM	May have increased salivation, nystagmus, dissociative state
Clonidine	4 mcg/kg PO 2 mcg/kg IN 2–4 mcg/kg IM	May affect seizure quality
Dexmedetomidine	0.5 mcg/kg IV 1–2 mcg/kg IN	May lower propofol dose requirement May be useful for treatment-resistant agitation following ECT
Midazolam	0.025 mg/kg IV	Likely to affect seizure quality Low dose may lead to paradoxic reactions May also be useful for treatment-resistant agitation following ECT
Diazepam	0.04–0.2 mg/kg IV/IM	Likely to affect seizure quality/duration
Lorazepam	0.05–0.2 mg/kg IV or PO	Likely to affect seizure quality/duration

Abbreviations: IV, intravenous; IM, intramuscular; IN, intranasal; PO, by mouth.

reserved before patient arrival, particularly if there is a potential for verbal or physical outbursts from the patient.

Benzodiazepines

An oral benzodiazepine, such as midazolam (0.5–0.75 mg/kg PO), is frequently prescribed to children in the preprocedural period before surgical procedures but must be used more judiciously in children presenting for ECT. Midazolam is a short-acting benzodiazepine with rapid onset of action and results in anxiolysis, muscle relaxation, anticonvulsant activity, and generation of anterograde amnesia. Like other benzodiazepines, midazolam facilitates the actions of gamma-aminobutyric acid (GABA) in the CNS. It binds to the benzodiazepine site on the GABA type A (GABA$_A$) receptor, thereby promoting the binding of GABA, enhancing its inhibitory activity in the CNS, and reducing the arousal of the cortical and limbic systems. Diazepam is a long-acting benzodiazepine, and lorazepam is an intermediate-acting benzodiazepine. Both of these agents have the same mechanism of action as midazolam but are less commonly used due to suppression of seizure duration. Benzodiazepines have consistently been shown to decrease the seizure duration and the therapeutic efficacy of both unilateral and bilateral ECT. A trial by Loimer and colleagues,[5] which compared the efficacy of intravenous midazolam with intravenous thiopental in adult ECT, was terminated early for ethical considerations because patients in the midazolam arm were unable to reach optimal seizure duration. Although low-dose intravenous midazolam (0.025 mg/kg) does not seem to prolong seizure duration over control, the ability of this dose to provide adequate preprocedural anxiolysis is unlikely and may result in paradoxic disinhibitory hyperactivity. Benzodiazepines may have some efficacy in the treatment of postictal delirium when administered in the recovery period as a single agent or when paired with droperidol.[6] Although the effect of oral preparations of benzodiazepines has not been studied in children undergoing ECT, routine premedication with benzodiazepines is likely not indicated and may result in a suboptimal treatment based on data from the adult population. Furthermore, some children may present for ECT on chronic benzodiazepine therapy, and a preprocedural discussion with the psychiatrist regarding optimal management of these patients is warranted.

Clonidine and Dexmedetomidine

Oral clonidine and intranasal dexmedetomidine are 2 options for premedication prescribed by some anesthesiologists. Clonidine is an alpha adrenergic agonist with higher selectivity for the alpha-2 receptor than alpha-1 receptors with an affinity predilection of 200:1. It acts centrally at the locus ceruleus but also has some peripheral effects. Dexmedetomidine is a highly selective alpha-2 adrenergic agonist with 8 times the affinity for alpha-2 adrenergic receptors when compared with clonidine. Data regarding the effects of clonidine on the quality of ECT are conflicting although dexmedetomidine does not seem to influence seizure duration. In addition, intravenous dexmedetomidine is useful in reducing postictal agitation and may slightly increase seizure duration when given before propofol.[7] Clonidine seems to be effective in blunting the hyperdynamic response to ECT although this issue may have little relevance in the pediatric population. These agents have not been studied in children undergoing ECT, but extrapolation of these data in adult patients suggest that dexmedetomidine may be an appropriate agent to facilitate separation of the child from family members and provide smooth induction conditions before ECT.

The hemodynamic consequences of ECT are typically more of a concern in the elderly patient with coronary artery disease, cardiac conduction disease, valvular disease, or ventricular dysfunction. These issues may be relevant to the child with preexisting cardiac dysfunction, although it must be noted that there are no reports of ECT performed on children with significant congenital or acquired cardiac disease. Bilateral ECT typically causes more cardiovascular effects than unilateral ECT. An initial, brief bradycardia may be observed with application of the stimulus due to greater parasympathetic outflow, but this is quickly replaced by a sustained sympathetic stimulation, which continues through the seizure and may persist for several minutes after cessation of EEG seizure activity. The increase in oxygen consumption, heart rate, and systemic blood pressure is usually well tolerated in healthy children. However, these issues, along with increases in pulmonary vascular resistance due to possible hypercapnia and hypoxia as a result of transient apnea may be extremely hazardous to children with septal defects, ventricular dysfunction, or those in the single ventricle palliation pathway. If the coexisting cardiac disease is significant, a multidisciplinary discussion between the anesthesiologist, psychiatrist, and cardiologist about the risks and benefits of proceeding with ECT should occur before treatment.

Procedural Considerations

The choice of hypnotic induction agent to be used before skeletal muscle relaxation is often debated. The anesthesiologist weighs the effects of various induction agents on induced seizure quality, while also taking into consideration the cardiopulmonary side effects of the agent, the child's comorbidities, and the recovery profile of the chosen agent. It is unclear if the seizure duration during ECT is directly related to the efficacy of the treatment, although seizure duration of less than 15 seconds is generally thought to be suboptimal. The induction agents listed later are all appropriate for use in pediatric ECT, and the choice of agent must be tailored to the individual patient and clinical situation. However, suboptimal treatment or side effect with one agent should prompt consideration of another agent at subsequent treatment sessions. These drugs have not been studied in pediatric patients undergoing ECT and so these recommendations are extrapolated from studies involving adult patients and experience at the authors' institution (**Table 2**).

Table 2 Induction agents used for pediatric electroconvulsive therapy		
Agent	**Suggested Dose and Route**	**Comments**
Methohexital	1–2 mg/kg IV	Dose-dependent decrease in motor and EEG seizure duration
Propofol	0.75–1.5 mg/kg IV	Shorter seizure activity but equivocal clinical outcomes; improved CV stability; quicker emergence; less PONV
Sevoflurane	6%–8% inspired concentration for induction; 1%–2% thereafter	Extra equipment required; more time-consuming
Thiopental	2–5 mg/kg IV	Shorter duration of seizure activity; risk for arrhythmias
Etomidate	0.15–0.3 mg/kg IV	Prolonged seizure duration; more hemodynamic instability and nausea/vomiting
Ketamine	0.7–2.8 mg/kg IV	Helpful for resistant seizures; reduced CV stability, possible increase in ICP
Succinylcholine	0.5–1.5 mg/kg IV	Avoid in neuroleptic malignant syndrome
Rocuronium	0.4–1.2 mg/kg IV	Does not cause hyperkalemia; requires reversal of neuromuscular blockade with sugammadex or neostigmine

Abbreviations: CV, cardiovascular; ICP, intracranial pressure; PONV, postoperative nausea and vomiting.

METHOHEXITAL

Methohexital is an ultrashort-acting barbiturate that is likely the most commonly used induction agent for ECTs in both the adult and pediatric population worldwide. Methohexital binds at a distinct chloride ionophore at the $GABA_A$ receptor, increasing the time the lithium ionophore is in the open position, prolonging the inhibitory effect of GABA in the thalamus. In addition, it also decreases glutamate responses. This agent may not be readily available at all institutions, because it is not commonly used for induction of anesthesia for other procedures. Methohexital (1–2 mg/kg intravenous [IV] bolus) has minimal effects on seizure duration as compared with other barbiturates that have more potent anticonvulsant properties. When a single induction dose is administered IV to children, the time to clinical recovery is 5 to 15 minutes, considerably shorter than other barbiturates such as thiopental. If seizure duration is thought to be the marker for successful ECT therapy, methohexital induction tends to provide the greatest seizure duration in most studies comparing this short-acting agent with others while also providing stable hemodynamics and a favorable recovery profile. Superiority of methohexital to other agents in the maintenance of seizure duration is clearly dose related, because a higher induction dosage tends to shorten seizure duration.[8]

Ketamine

Intramuscular ketamine (5–10 mg/kg IM) is very effective as premedication for the especially anxious, fearful, or combative child. Ketamine acts as a selective antagonist of the N-methyl-D-aspartate receptor, which is a glutamate receptor and ion channel protein found in neurons. Ketamine also has interactions at the opioid, monoaminergic, muscarinic, and voltage sensitive calcium ion channels. Unlike other anesthetic agents, ketamine does not interact with GABA receptors. Ketamine is generally considered a second-line induction agent behind methohexital for ECT, but its properties are quite clinically favorable for this procedure. Ketamine lowers the seizure threshold and has shown greater seizure duration with increased amplitude when compared with methohexital.[9] Indeed, intravenous induction with ketamine (1–3 mg/kg IV) may be indicated when standard methohexital therapy results in a suboptimal treatment. There is also recent interest in ketamine as treatment for refractory depression and so this agent may serve a dual purpose in certain patient populations.[10] The major drawbacks of ketamine anesthesia for pediatric ECT are hallucinatory effects extending into the postoperative period and prolonged recovery times. Although this incidence has not been studied in the pediatric population, this may be significant given the dose required for induction of general anesthesia before muscle relaxation and the short duration of the procedure. Theoretically, ketamine-related catecholamine release paired with the sympathetic response associated with ECT might cause cardiac compromise in the child with significant cardiovascular comorbidities. For pediatric ECT, ketamine is likely the second most appropriate intravenous induction agent if methohexital is unavailable or contraindicated given its ability to facilitate favorable ECT conditions.

Propofol

Propofol has recently gained greater acceptance as an anesthetic induction agent in adults receiving ECT. Propofol is a dialkylphenol (2,6, diisopropylphenol) that potentiates the inhibitory function of GABA and directly activates $GABA_A$ receptor function. Sensitivity of the $GABA_A$ receptor to propofol is thought to be secondary to alpha, beta, and gamma subunits interacting with the drug. Propofol also interacts with various other neurotransmitter receptors such as glycine, nicotinic, and M1 muscarinic receptors. Propofol is far more readily available and familiar to the modern anesthesiologist than barbiturates, and there have been more studies that compare its effects to the "gold standard" of methohexital than any other agent. Propofol has potent anticonvulsant properties at dosages commonly used for induction of general anesthesia (1.5–2.5 mg/kg IV for adolescents), and this dose may significantly affect the quality of treatment, although data are conflicting.[11] These effects are likely dose dependent, because a minimally hypnotic dose (0.75 mg/kg) provides seizure duration that is similar to a standard dose of methohexital. Propofol anesthesia does not provide earlier emergence times or faster recovery periods. When compared with methohexital, propofol seems to cause fewer cardiac arrhythmias and its potent cardiac depressant effects seem to mitigate the hyperdynamic response to ECT. Although these effects may be important for adults with preexisting cardiac conditions, specifically coronary artery disease, these cardiovascular benefits are unlikely to be clinically relevant in the pediatric population. There is some evidence that propofol requirements increase with subsequent ECT sessions. However, this has been disputed with follow-up studies, and the phenomenon is not witnessed when propofol is used as an induction agent for other procedures. Propofol is likely the third-line intravenous agent for pediatric ECT if methohexital or ketamine are unavailable or contraindicated provided that the lowest possible dose to produce clinical effect is used.

Sevoflurane

Inhalational induction of general anesthesia with volatile anesthetic gases is commonly performed for younger children before obtaining intravenous access.[12] The mechanism by which fluorinated isopropyl ethers, such as sevoflurane, produce a state of general anesthesia is yet to be fully elucidated despite decades of study. There is agreement that volatile anesthetics induce general anesthesia by enhancing inhibitory pathways and attenuating excitatory channels in the brain. Sevoflurane is believed to directly activate GABA receptors, alter the release and reuptake of neurotransmitters at postsynaptic terminals, and/or alter ionic conductance through neuronal membranes. Sevoflurane induction for ECT provides adequate conditions for treatment and provides a solid option for anesthesiologists who are comfortable and experienced with this anesthetic technique.[12] Sevoflurane inhalational induction has been compared with methohexital and propofol intravenous induction in clinical trials with mixed, but overall favorable, comparative results in terms of seizure dynamics and safety.[13] However, inhalational induction takes longer to reach anesthetic depth sufficient for treatment and also leads to slightly longer recovery periods. Utilization of volatile anesthetics requires an anesthesia machine and vaporizer, which may increase the complexity and costs over intravenous induction techniques. This may also preclude the performance of ECT at locations remote to the operating room in many institutions. For pediatric ECT, sevoflurane inhalational induction is a very reasonable option but remains suboptimal to the process of intravenous induction with methohexital, ketamine, or propofol. Nitrous oxide is often administered concomitantly with sevoflurane to hasten the induction sequence by imparting complex second gas and concentrating effects. After induction with 8% sevoflurane in a nitrous oxide/oxygen mix, it is prudent to terminate nitrous oxide flows, ventilate with 100% oxygen, and decrease the sevoflurane vaporizer output to 1.1% to 1.3% at the time of stimulus to provide the most favorable conditions for ECT.[14] Intravenous access should be placed after inhalational induction to appropriately treat potential complications such as laryngospasm or ECT-induced arrhythmias.

Thiopental

Thiopental is an ultrashort-acting barbiturate with anesthetic activity that enhances the inhibitory actions of $GABA_A$ in the brain by binding to the $GABA_A$/chloride ionophore receptor complex. Binding causes decreased excitability of neurons and synaptic inhibition, leading to general anesthesia. Both methohexital and thiopental have had periods of unavailability in the United States, and the overall usage of barbiturates for the induction of anesthesia is decreasing worldwide. However, thiopental (1.5–2.5 mg/kg IV bolus) is likely the more commonly available and familiar drug to anesthesiologists. Investigations into the effects of both agents on seizure duration have yielded mixed results. The most commonly cited article is by Mokriski and colleagues,[15] which demonstrated that methohexital prolonged seizure duration by greater than 5 seconds when compared with thiopental. Thiopental has also been criticized for its potential to induce arrhythmias, specifically premature ventricular contractions, and methohexital seems to be safer in this aspect. However, additional comparative studies are difficult to compare due to the variations in induction dosages between studies. A recent retrospective review article that examined nearly 100 adult patients receiving ECT showed that there was no improvement in outcome or Global Assessment of Functioning scores when methohexital was used over thiopental. For pediatric ECT, thiopental is suboptimal to methohexital induction. Thiopental is likely suboptimal to propofol, ketamine, and sevoflurane as well and so should be reserved for the rare case in which these agents are unavailable or contraindicated.

Etomidate

Etomidate is an imidazole derivative with short-acting anesthetic properties. Its effects are secondary to interactions with the $GABA_A$ receptor, which enhance the inhibitory effect of GABA on the CNS. It also plays a role in benzodiazepine binding at the $GABA_A$ receptor site. Induction of anesthesia with etomidate (0.15–0.3 mg/kg IV bolus) has consistently been shown to prolong seizure duration when compared with methohexital, propofol, and thiopental. Etomidate also tends to have less cardiac depressant effects, which may be of some benefit in children with depressed cardiac contractility who present for ECT. Etomidate, like ketamine, is unlikely to be a first-line agent due to its side-effect profile but may be useful in pediatric patients undergoing ECT with suboptimal prior treatments with seizure durations of less than 20 seconds. Side effects of postprocedural nausea and emesis, postictal agitation/confusion, and adrenal suppression are significant problems with this agent.

Opioids

Opioids are a group of commonly used analgesic agents that bind 4 distinct classes of opioid receptors. Different opioids can act as agonists, antagonists, or partial agonists depending on the specific G protein–coupled opioid receptor to which they bind. Clinically, analgesia is mostly due to opioid agonists binding to mu receptors. The major opioid that has been used in the anesthetic management of ECT is remifentanil (0.001 mg/kg IV bolus). Although there are no pediatric studies evaluating the use of remifentanil, this ultrashort-acting opioid analgesic is typically used in combination with intravenous hypnotic agents or inhaled sevoflurane.[16] Remifentanil may indirectly improve the seizure quality and duration during ECT. Remifentanil, given along with a hypnotic in the induction sequence, will reduce the inherent anticonvulsant activity of the hypnotic itself, because less hypnotic agent is required to induce general anesthesia. Because of rapid extrahepatic metabolism of remifentanil by nonspecific esterases, the context-sensitive half time after termination is 3 minutes, largely independent of infusion duration.

Succinylcholine

Induction of the electrical stimulus for ECT is followed by vigorous motor seizure activity, which is typically mitigated by administration of a muscle relaxant after induction of anesthesia. If muscle relaxation is not administered, the ability of the patient to sustain injury is significant as severe joint dislocation and even hip fracture has been reported during ECT-induced seizure. Classically, the depolarizing muscle relaxant succinylcholine has been used due to its rapid onset, profound muscle relaxation, and fastest recovery profile. The effective dose of succinylcholine for ECT has been debated. Despite the Royal College of Psychiatrists' recommendation of 0.5 mg/kg IV bolus, the clinically appropriate dose for children is likely higher at 0.75 to 1.5 mg/kg IV bolus because of a larger volume of distribution.[17] Children who present with an elevated serum potassium level, have risk factors for developing malignant hyperthermia, or have a history of significant succinylcholine induced myalgias may require a nondepolarizing neuromuscular blocking agent such as cisatracurium, vecuronium, or rocuronium to provide muscle relaxation.[18] Children treated with dopamine-depleting medications (such as antipsychotics) may develop neuroleptic malignant syndrome (NMS), which is characterized by the triad of altered mental status, fever, and muscle rigidity. This entity confers high mortality if not identified and treated early. ECT is a potential treatment for refractory NMS due to its ability to increase CNS dopamine levels, but succinylcholine must be used with caution given the potential of hyperkalemia due to rhabdomyolysis.[19]

Rocuronium

Because of the brevity of the ECT procedure, the administration of nondepolarizing muscle relaxants may require intubation, a brief period of mechanical ventilation, reversal with an anticholinesterase agent, or administration of sugammadex, which significantly increases the risk associated with this procedure and must be discussed during the informed consent process. If the patient has a contraindication to succinylcholine, the nondepolarizing neuromuscular blocking agent rocuronium is an excellent alternative. Rocuronium has a rapid onset of action, and the neuromuscular blockade conferred by this agent may immediately be terminated with sugammadex if required. Rocuronium is an aminosteroid neuromuscular-blocking agent and, like other nondepolarizing neuromuscular blocking agents, acts by competitively binding to nicotinic cholinergic receptors at the motor end plate. Binding of rocuronium blocks acetylcholine from binding to these receptors preventing depolarization and subsequent skeletal muscle contraction. The nondepolarizing neuromuscular blocking agents do not cause hyperkalemia and can be given safely to patients susceptible to malignant hyperthermia. The dose to achieve intubating conditions for a standard induction in pediatric patients is 0.6 mg/kg IV bolus with a time to onset of 3 minutes. A higher dose of 1.2 mg/kg IV bolus may be used to achieve intubating conditions within 60 seconds. To facilitate adequate return of respiratory muscle function, the neuromuscular blockade must be reversed using either neostigmine or sugammadex. Although rare, allergic reactions leading to anaphylaxis can occur with rocuronium at rates similar to other neuromuscular-blocking agents.

Sugammadex

Sugammadex is the first clinically available drug in the new class of selective relaxant-binding agents (SRBA). It reverses neuromuscular blocking action by selectively binding aminosteroid nondepolarizing muscle relaxants such as rocuronium or vecuronium. Sugammadex is a modified, anionic gamma cyclodextrin derivative containing a hydrophilic exterior and a hydrophobic core. On intravenous administration, negatively charged portions of the sugammadex molecule selectively and reversibly bind to positively charged portions of the muscle relaxant. At proper doses, it is able to reverse any depth of neuromuscular block conferred by rocuronium or vecuronium. Rocuronium, when used with sugammadex, is slowly becoming the "gold standard" muscle relaxant for rapid sequence induction of general anesthesia and for procedures of short duration requiring muscle relaxation. Despite the unavailability of long-term data regarding their use, the pharmacologic profile of SRBAs could make them a mainstay for use in ECT.

Postprocedural Considerations

ECT is a safe outpatient procedure in children with minimal comorbidities. Standard postprocedural criteria for discharge from the recovery area such as stable cardiopulmonary status and adequate oral intake should be followed per the institution's policies. Although neurologic complications are uncommon, it is important to note a child's return to baseline neurologic status after ECT. Minor postictal delirium or agitation may respond to midazolam or small doses of propofol.[20] The extreme increase in cerebral blood flow as a result of sympathetic stimulation has been associated with intracranial hemorrhage. Although short-term cognitive dysfunction is not uncommon after ECT, any such deficits should be documented and noted during presentation for the next subsequent treatment. Administration of an antiemetic may be advisable especially if agents with greater emetic potential, such as sevoflurane and etomidate, are used. Succinylcholine-related myalgia, which is unlikely to be dose related, responds well to nonsteroidal antiinflammatory agents such as ketorolac (**Table 3**).

Table 3
Adjuncts used for pediatric electroconvulsive therapy

Agent	Suggested Dose and Route	Comments
Midazolam	0.05–0.1 mg/kg IV	Termination of prolonged seizure Treatment of postictal agitation
Diazepam	0.1–0.2 mg/kg IV	Termination of prolonged seizure Treatment of postictal agitation
Ondansetron	0.1 mg/kg IV	Antiemetic
Ketorolac	0.5 mg/kg IV	Reduction of myalgias

SUMMARY

ECT is a safe and effective tool for the treatment of a variety of pediatric and adolescent psychiatric disorders as well as in the treatment of pediatric refractory status epilepticus. Anesthesia for the child undergoing ECT should ideally provide deep hypnosis, ensure muscle relaxation to reduce injury, have minimal effect on seizure dynamics, and allow for rapid recovery to baseline neurologic and cardiopulmonary status. Multiple anesthetic agents are acceptable for use during ECT and the choice of specific agents should factor in the patient's underlying comorbidities and desired recovery profile.

REFERENCES

1. Hooten WM, Rasmussen KG Jr. Effects of general anesthetic agents in adults receiving electroconvulsive therapy: a systematic review. J ECT 2008;24(3): 208–23.
2. Poole KA, Weber N, Aziz M. Case report: quetiapine and refractory hypotension during general anesthesia in the operating room. Anesth Analg 2013;117(3):641–3.
3. Ding Z, White PF. Anesthesia for electroconvulsive therapy. Anesth Analg 2002; 94(5):1351–64.
4. Kranaster L, Hoyer C, Janke C, et al. Bispectral index monitoring and seizure quality optimization in electroconvulsive therapy. Pharmacopsychiatry 2013; 46(4):147–50.
5. Loimer N, Hofmann P, Chaudhry HR. Midazolam shortens seizure duration following electroconvulsive therapy. J Psychiatr Res 1992;26(2):97–101.
6. Hines AH, Labbate LA. Combination midazolam and droperidol for severe post-ECT agitation. Convuls Ther 1997;13(2):113–4.
7. O'Brien EM, Rosenquist PB, Kimball JN, et al. Dexmedetomidine and the successful management of electroconvulsive therapy postictal agitation: a case report. J ECT 2010;26(2):131–3.
8. Avramov MN, Husain MM, White PF. The comparative effects of methohexital, propofol, and etomidate for electroconvulsive therapy. Anesth Analg 1995; 81(3):596–602.
9. Staton RD, Enderle JD, Gerst JW. The electroencephalographic pattern during electroconvulsive therapy. IV. Spectral energy distributions with methohexital, innovar and ketamine anesthesias. Clin Electroencephalogr 1986;17(4):203–15.
10. Lee EE, Della Selva MP, Liu A, et al. Ketamine as a novel treatment for major depressive disorder and bipolar depression: a systematic review and quantitative meta-analysis. Gen Hosp Psychiatry 2015;37(2):178–84.

11. Geretsegger C, Nickel M, Judendorfer B, et al. Propofol and methohexital as anesthetic agents for electroconvulsive therapy: a randomized, double-blind comparison of electroconvulsive therapy seizure quality, therapeutic efficacy, and cognitive performance. J ECT 2007;23(4):239–43.

12. Calarge CA, Crowe RR, Gergis SD, et al. The comparative effects of sevoflurane and methohexital for electroconvulsive therapy. J ECT 2003;19(4):221–5.

13. Hodgson RE, Dawson P, Hold AR, et al. Anaesthesia for electroconvulsive therapy: a comparison of sevoflurane with propofol. Anaesth Intensive Care 2004; 32(2):241–5.

14. Rasmussen KG, Laurila DR, Brady BM, et al. Anesthesia outcomes in a randomized double-blind trial of sevoflurane and thiopental for induction of general anesthesia in electroconvulsive therapy. J ECT 2007;23(4):236–8.

15. Mokriski BK, Nagle SE, Papuchis GC, et al. Electroconvulsive therapy-induced cardiac arrhythmias during anesthesia with methohexital, thiamylal, or thiopental sodium. J Clin Anesth 1992;4(3):208–12.

16. Ulusoy H, Cekic B, Besir A, et al. Sevoflurane/remifentanil versus propofol/remifentanil for electroconvulsive therapy: comparison of seizure duration and haemodynamic responses. J Int Med Res 2014;42(1):111–9.

17. Fredman B, Smith I, d'Etienne J, et al. Use of muscle relaxants for electroconvulsive therapy: how much is enough? Anesth Analg 1994;78(1):195–6.

18. Mirzakhani H, Guchelaar HJ, Welch CA, et al. Minimum effective doses of succinylcholine and rocuronium during electroconvulsive therapy: a prospective, randomized, crossover trial. Anesth Analg 2016;123(3):587–96.

19. Koster TD, Kooistra WE, Tuinman AG. Near miss with succinylcholine for electroconvulsive therapy: a case report. Eur J Anaesthesiol 2014;31(8):441–3.

20. O'Reardon JP, Takieddine N, Datto CJ, et al. Propofol for the management of emergence agitation after electroconvulsive therapy: review of a case series. J ECT 2006;22(4):247–52.

Transcranial Magnetic Stimulation for Adolescent Depression

Paul E. Croarkin, DO, MS[a],*, Frank P. MacMaster, PhD[b]

KEYWORDS

- Adolescent • Brain stimulation • Depression • GABA • Glutamate
- Neuromodulation • Transcranial magnetic stimulation • TMS

KEY POINTS

- Adolescent depression is a substantial global public health problem, which contributes to academic failure, occupational impairment, deficits in social function, substance use disorders, teen pregnancy, and completed suicide.
- Existing treatment approaches, such as psychotherapy, pharmacotherapy, or combination treatment, often have suboptimal results and uncertain safety profiles.
- Brain stimulation modalities, such as transcranial magnetic stimulation, have the potential for enduring, brain-based interventions for adolescents with depression.
- Existing work with transcranial magnetic stimulation in adolescents is nascent and larger, developmentally informed studies are needed.
- Treatment with transcranial magnetic stimulation may address imbalances in cortical GABAergic and glutamatergic neural circuitry.

Disclosure Statement: Dr P.E. Croarkin has received research grant support from Pfizer, National Institute of Mental Health, the Brain and Behavior Research Foundation, and the Mayo Clinic Foundation. He has served as a site subprincipal or principal investigator (without additional compensation) for Eli Lilly and Co, Forest Laboratories, Inc, Merck & Co, Inc, and Pfizer, Inc; has received equipment support from Neuronetics, Inc; and receives supplies and genotyping services from Assurex Health, Inc for an investigator-initiated study. He is the primary investigator for a multicenter study funded by Neuronetics, Inc. He is a site investigator for a study funded by NeoSync, Inc. Dr F.P. MacMaster has received research grant support from the Canadian Institutes of Health Research, the Canadian Foundation for Innovation, Branch Out Neurologic Foundation, Alberta Health Services, and the Alberta Children's Hospital Foundation.
[a] Child and Adolescent Psychiatry, Mayo Clinic College of Medicine and Science, 200 First Street Southwest, Rochester, MN 55905, USA; [b] Strategic Clinical Network for Addictions and Mental Health, University of Calgary, Alberta Children's Hospital, Office Number: B4-511, 2500 University Dr. NWCalgary, Alberta, T2N 1N4, Canada
* Corresponding author.
E-mail address: croarkin.paul@mayo.edu

Child Adolesc Psychiatric Clin N Am 28 (2019) 33–43
https://doi.org/10.1016/j.chc.2018.07.003
1056-4993/19/© 2018 Elsevier Inc. All rights reserved.

INTRODUCTION

Adolescent major depressive disorder (MDD) is a major public health problem with a lifetime prevalence estimated as high as 14% to 20% in epidemiologic studies.[1] Worldwide, MDD is a leading cause of disease burden.[2,3] Adolescent depression frequently involves a profound biologic component and ensuing delayed recovery, frequent recurrences, comorbidity, substance abuse, and increased risk for suicide.[1,4] Initial management of moderate to severe MDD in adolescents involves treatment with psychotherapy and selective serotonin reuptake inhibitors (SSRIs).[5,6] Remission rates and outcomes are often poor because this treatment does not target relevant, underlying adolescent pathophysiology.[5,7] Ongoing controversy regarding the effectiveness and safety of SSRIs in young individuals underscores the importance for an improved understanding of the biological mechanisms involved in adolescent depression.[8,9] Finally, access to evidence based psychotherapy is often limited.[10]

Transcranial magnetic stimulation (TMS) has increasingly been considered an investigational treatment for adolescents with depression who do not respond to standard treatment modalities, such as cognitive behavioral therapy and SSRIs.[11,12] Treatment with TMS involves the stimulation of cortical neurons with magnetic pulses and is now widely available as a clinical treatment for adults. Current US Food and Drug Administration–cleared TMS treatments involve 5 daily treatments per week, for 4 to 6 weeks, with 10-Hz, 120% motor threshold stimulation applied to the left dorsolateral prefrontal cortex (LDLPFC).[13–15] Early adolescent research was informed by this approach, but there is a formidable parameter space (for example, coil location, frequency, intensity, duration of treatment, concurrent interventions, and brain state during treatment) to consider for TMS treatment.[16,17] The heterogeneity of depression in adolescents arguably presents an added layer of complexity.[1,16,18]

TYPES OF TRANSCRANIAL MAGNETIC STIMULATION

Early therapeutic TMS research and clinical practice for depression in adults have largely used low-frequency (1 Hz) or high-frequency (5–20 Hz) stimulation over the dorsolateral prefrontal cortex.[13,19] There have been a variety of variations in dosing with time to include deep TMS, accelerated protocols, synchronized TMS, priming protocols, and patterned stimulation.[20] More contemporary work has examined theta burst stimulation (TBS) dosing strategies as potentially more efficient and durable pulse sequences for the modification of cortical activity.[21] Treatment with TBS holds the promise of reducing the time burden of treatment for patients. TBS sequences deliver groups of 3 high-frequency pulses (50 Hz) with interstimulus intervals of 200 ms (5 Hz). There are 2 primary TBS patterns that are thought to have discordant neurophysiologic effects.[21,22] Continuous theta burst stimulation (cTBS) involves the delivery of TBS pulses without interruption (typically 20–40 seconds 300–600 pulses) and is thought to decrease cortical excitability.[22] Intermittent theta burst stimulation (iTBS) delivers 2-second trains of TBS (30 pulses) every 10 seconds and is thought to increase cortical excitability.[22,23] Recent work in adults with treatment-resistant depression suggests that iTBS may be equivalent to standard 10-Hz repetitive theta burst stimulation (rTMS) in terms of effectiveness, safety, and tolerability.[24]

STUDIES OF TRANSCRANIAL MAGNETIC STIMULATION IN DEPRESSED ADOLESCENTS

Table 1 summarizes existing therapeutic studies of TMS for adolescents with depression. At present, there are 10 publications describing the treatment of 112 unique

Table 1
Summary of therapeutic transcranial magnetic stimulation studies for adolescent depression

References	N	Mean Age (y)	Frequency	Intensity (%)	Location	Clinical Outcome
Walter et al,[25] 2001	4	16	1–10 Hz (variable)	90–110	LDLPFC	2 responders (one nonresponder had bipolar depression)
Loo et al,[26] 2006	2	16	10 Hz	110	LDLPFC	2 responders
Bloch et al,[27] 2008	9	17	10 Hz	80	LDLPFC	3 responders 1 partial responder
Wall et al,[28] 2011	8	16	10 Hz	120	LDLPFC	6 responders
Mayer et al,[29] 2012 (3-y follow-up from Bloch et al,[27] 2008 study)	8	17	10 Hz	80	LDLPFC	Improvement in depressive symptoms was durable at follow-up
Le et al,[30] 2013	25	11	1 Hz	110	SMA	Group level improvement in depressive symptoms
Yang et al,[31] 2014	6	18	10 Hz	120	LDLPFC	4 responders
Wall et al,[12] 2016	10	15	10 Hz	120	LDLPFC	6 responders
Farzan et al,[32] 2017	16	21	iTBS and cTBS	80	LDLPFC (iTBS) RDLPFC (cTBS)	4 responders 9 partial responders
MacMaster et al,[33] 2018	32	17	10 Hz	120	LDLPFC	18 responders

Abbreviations: RDLPFC, right dorsolateral prefrontal cortex; SMA, supplementary motor area.

participants.[12,25–33] Existing literature is almost entirely composed of case reports and open-label studies. The 2006 study by Loo and colleagues[26] describes a randomized controlled trial. However, the results from 2 participants assigned to active TMS treatment are all that is described in the publication.[26] The study by Le and colleagues[30] describes the treatment of 25 children with Tourette syndrome. These participants did not have a diagnosis of MDD at baseline. However, depressive symptoms were tracked and demonstrated group level improvement over the course of TMS treatment.[30] This study is also unique and important to consider because it examined 1-Hz TMS, which has not been adequately studied in child and adolescent populations with psychiatric disorders.[11] Otherwise, most studies examined 10-Hz TMS sessions with protocols adapted from landmark adult studies of TMS.[12,14,15,26–28,31,34] Farzan and colleagues[32] have pioneered work with iTBS in adolescents and young adults. Given the increased efficiency of iTBS in terms of both delivery and potential impact on synaptic plasticity, this line of research is critical for future optimization of TMS protocols involving adolescents.[32,35]

SAFETY

Systematic data on the safety of TMS in children and adolescent are lacking.[11,36] Although generally considered safe, TMS interventions could have divergent tolerability and safety profiles across various stages of neurodevelopment. Common concerns include the rare risk of seizure induction, adverse neurocognitive effects, new or exacerbated psychiatric symptoms (such as increased suicidality, hypomania, or mania), aberrant alterations in neuroplasticity, and pain related to the procedure.[36] Recent, erudite commentaries have highlighted these concerns and the depth of existing knowledge gaps.[37,38]

Krishnan and colleagues[36] recently reviewed existing literature focused on both TMS and transcranial current stimulation. The review included data from 35 publications focused on the use of TMS in children and adolescents 3 to 18 years of age. There were very few reported adverse events or tolerability problems among the 322 participants undergoing TMS procedures. Four of these participants (1.2%) had a major negative side effect. Two participants (0.62%) had a seizure, and 2 other participants had syncopal episodes (0.62%). Minor side effects such as headache (11.5%) and scalp pain (2.5%) were described as short lived and typically resolved without intervention or with the use of over-the-counter nonsteroidal anti-inflammatory drugs. Other reported adverse events included musculoskeletal problems, twitching, and fatigue. These effects were described as mild and transitory. These data are encouraging and suggest that TMS is relatively safe and tolerable in children and adolescents with appropriate precautions. However, existing work also underscores that in most instances, systematic adverse effect and tolerability data from TMS exposure in children and adolescents are not collected. Systematic, long-term, follow-up studies are also lacking.[36]

The clinical effects and safety of TMS have been examined in numerous other publications.[20] Published guidelines have been successful in ensuring subject safety.[13,39,40] In most cases, TMS cannot be applied to individuals with metal in their head (except the mouth). The greatest safety concern is the potential of inducing a seizure. The risk of this is small even with rTMS. The incidence of this has been estimated as no greater than 0.1% to 0.6% (or 1–6 in 1000), which is comparable to the incidence of spontaneous seizures in patients taking antidepressant medications.[41] In cases in which seizures have been induced in participants, these individuals have recovered with no recurrences.[36,39,42] There are 3 prior reported seizures in adolescents receiving TMS.[43–45] In 2 instances the participants were concurrently taking epileptogenic medications (sertraline and olanzapine).[43,44] One of these participants had also consumed large amounts of alcohol before the TMS session (a reported 0.20% blood alcohol level 30 minutes after the seizure).[43] In another instance, a depressed patient with no risk factors had a seizure with the application of deep TMS.[45] Presently, it is not clear if the risk for seizure induction during TMS with adolescents is different from that of adults.[42]

RECENT STUDIES

In 2015, NeuroStar Advanced Therapy launched the largest, randomized controlled trial of TMS for adolescents (12–21 years of age) with MDD to date.[46] This trial is scheduled to conclude in late 2018 and will examine the safety and efficacy of Neuro-Star TMS in approximately 100 adolescent participants. The protocol is a randomized, sham-controlled, triple-masked design for the acute treatment of MDD, with a subsequent open-label phase and posttreatment follow-up study. Eligible patients are adolescents aged 12 to 21 with MDD that has failed to respond to at least 1 but not more than 4 prior antidepressant trials. Phase I offers 6 weeks of either active 10-Hz TMS or sham treatment applied to the LDLPFC. Phase II provides 6 weeks of open-label 10-Hz TMS to patients who did not receive protocol-defined clinical benefit in phase I. Patients with protocol-defined clinical benefit in phase I or II are eligible for phase III, a 6-month follow-up study that provides re-treatment with TMS for the reemergence of depressive symptoms. The protocol and study will provide the largest data set to date for the examination of tolerability, safety, and clinical effects of 10-Hz TMS for MDD in adolescents.[46]

FUTURE DIRECTIONS

Neurostimulation technologies such as TMS have great potential as enduring, brain-based interventions for depression in adolescents.[11,35] Treatment with rTMS likely addresses pathologic imbalances in cortical GABAergic inhibitory and excitatory glutamatergic frontolimbic neurocircuitry.[35,47] However, at present, there are many unknowns regarding optimal stimulation parameters and potential biomarkers for depressed adolescents receiving TMS.[11,16] Later this year, a National Institute of Mental Health–funded, dose-finding, biomarker validation, and effectiveness study of 1–Hz versus 10-Hz TMS for adolescents with depression will begin enrollment with the aim of addressing these questions (NIMH R01MH113700).[48]

Imbalances in GABAergic and glutamatergic tone play a key role in depression,[49,50] pathophysiologic stress responses,[51,52] and emotional numbing or anhedonia found in behavioral manifestations of the negative valence system.[53] These GABAergic and glutamatergic imbalances have differential causes, effects, and behavioral manifestations in adolescents as compared with adults.[49,53–56] For example, recent preclinical work has demonstrated that repeated stress in adolescent rats inhibits GABAergic projections to the amygdala, thereby impairing regulatory neurocircuitry.[57] In adult rats, chronic stress facilitates glutamatergic excitatory neurotransmission with ensuing effects on the lateral nucleus of the amygdala, hippocampus, and frontal cortex.[57–61] Developmental differences in frontolimbic GABAergic and glutamatergic tone may underlie variances in adolescent depressive symptom presentations and treatment responsivity.[53,61] A deeper understanding of frontolimbic GABAergic and glutamatergic tone in adolescent depression would assist with precision medicine approaches and intervention development.[16] TMS and magnetic resonance spectroscopy (MRS) provide complementary measures or cortical GABAergic and glutamategeric tone.[62–65] Single- and paired-pulse TMS paradigms are used to study the physiology of the brain. Neurophysiologic measures collected with TMS, such as intracortical facilitation (ICF), short-interval intracortical inhibition (SICI), long-interval intracortical inhibition (LICI), and the cortical silent period (CSP), are noninvasive measures of cortical GABAergic and glutamatergic tone.[64–66] Prior work suggests that ICF is a valid marker of glutamatergic tone, and it may have utility as a biomarker for depression in adolescents.[55,67] Ultra-high-field, 7 T MRS adequately quantifies GABA, glutamate, and glutamine concentrations in the cortex for complementary data examining GABAergic and glutamatergic tone.[68] Concurrent measures with TMS neurophysiologic paradigms and 7 T MRS would provide a refined understanding of GABAergic and glutamatergic tone in disorders of the negative valence systems and mechanistic studies of brain stimulation treatments such as TMS.[68,69]

Fig. 1 summarized the protocol of the pending study. Participants in phase I will be stratified based on ICF testing (high or low) at baseline. An ICF of greater than 1.5 at baseline is considered "high" and an ICF ≤1.5 is considered "low." After stratification, adolescents are randomized to either LDLPFC 1-Hz rTMS with 2400 continuous pulses per session at 120% motor threshold or LDLPFC 10-Hz rTMS with 4 seconds on 36 seconds off for 2400 pulses each session at 120% of resting motor threshold. Hence sessions in each treatment arm with 2 different types of rTMS (1 Hz and 10 Hz) will have identical intensities (120% motor threshold), durations (40 minutes), number of pulses (2400), and treatment location (LDLPFC). Participant nonresponders in phase I will be offered the opportunity to enroll in a phase II. Participants will be

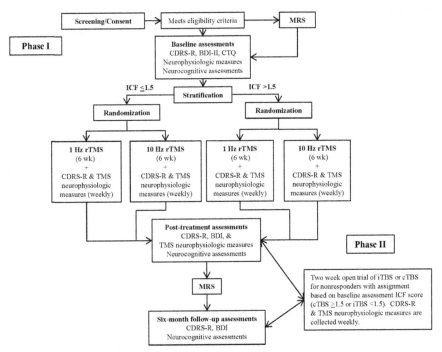

Fig. 1. Study schema. BDI, Beck depression inventory; CDRS-R, children's depression rating scale-revised; cTBS, continuous theta burst stimulation; CTQ, childhood trauma questionnaire; Hz, hertz; ICF, intracortical facilitation; iTBS, intermittent theta burst stimulation; MRS, magnetic resonance spectroscopy; TMS, transcranial magnetic stimulation.

undergo therapeutic rTMS sessions with a Neurostar XPLOR system magnetic stimulator. The research team will localize rTMS treatment sites with the Beam F3 method.[70] Prior research demonstrates that this is a valid and reliable method for scalp location of the dorsolateral prefrontal cortex with comparable results to more expensive, time-intensive, MRI-guided approaches.[71] Prior research demonstrates that the Beam F3 method is a feasible and reliable method for rTMS treatment localization in adolescents.[12] Efficacy measures (Children's Depression Rating Scale Revised [CDRS-R])[72] and TMS biomarkers will be collected at baseline and weekly. The TMS biomarker panel includes ICF, Motor threshold (MT) SICI, LICI, and CSP. Adolescent participants receiving TMS will have the opportunity to undergo pre- and post-7-T MRS scans to collect cortical GABA, glutamate, and glutamine levels.[48]

Participants in phase II will be assigned to 2 weeks of cTBS if their ICF measure (baseline assessment for TBS extension trial) is >1.5. Participants will be assigned to 2 weeks of iTBS if their ICF (baseline assessment for TBS extension trial) is ≤1.5. Extension trial TBS will be applied to the LDLPFC with the Beam F3 method. Participants receiving cTBS will receive 10 daily (5 sessions per week for 2 weeks) 120-second trains of uninterrupted TBS for 1800 pulses at 80% motor threshold. Participants receiving iTBS will receive 10 daily (5 sessions per week for 2 weeks) 2-second trains every 10 seconds for a total of 570 seconds for 1800 pulses at 80% motor threshold. Efficacy measures (CDRS-R) and TMS biomarkers will be collected at baseline, 1 week, and 2 weeks. The TMS biomarker panel includes ICF, MT SICI, LICI, and CSP.[48]

SUMMARY

Safe, effective, brain-based treatments for depression in adolescents could alleviate substantial morbidity and mortality.[16] Early investigational TMS for adolescent depression is promising.[11,36] These data suggest that the clinical effects, safety, and tolerability of TMS in adolescents may be similar to what has been described in adults.[11,36] However, enthusiasm must be tempered by considerations for neurodevelopment and the unknowns associated with TMS exposure in adolescents.[16,37,38] Larger studies will soon provide more systematic data to examine the clinical tolerability, safety, and clinical effects of TMS in adolescents with depression.[46] Planned dose-finding and biomarker development studies hold the prospect of expanding the knowledge base of TMS use in depressed adolescents, the pathophysiology of depression in youth, and how TMS modulates cortical GABAergic and glutamatergic neurochemistry.[48]

REFERENCES

1. Thapar A, Collishaw S, Pine DS, et al. Depression in adolescence. Lancet 2012; 379(9820):1056–67.
2. Gore FM, Bloem PJ, Patton GC, et al. Global burden of disease in young people aged 10-24 years: a systematic analysis. Lancet 2011;377(9783):2093–102.
3. Whiteford HA, Degenhardt L, Rehm J, et al. Global burden of disease attributable to mental and substance use disorders: findings from the Global Burden of Disease Study 2010. Lancet 2013;382(9904):1575–86.
4. Naicker K, Galambos NL, Zeng Y, et al. Social, demographic, and health outcomes in the 10 years following adolescent depression. J Adolesc Health 2013;52(5):533–8.
5. March JS, Silva S, Petrycki S, et al. The treatment for adolescents with depression study (TADS): long-term effectiveness and safety outcomes. Arch Gen Psychiatry 2007;64(10):1132–43.

6. Kennard BD, Emslie GJ, Mayes TL, et al. Sequential treatment with fluoxetine and relapse–prevention CBT to improve outcomes in pediatric depression. Am J Psychiatry 2014;171(10):1083–90.

7. Walkup JT. Antidepressant efficacy for depression in children and adolescents: industry- and NIMH-funded studies. Am J Psychiatry 2017;174(5):430–7.

8. Hammad TA, Laughren T, Racoosin J. Suicidality in pediatric patients treated with antidepressant drugs. Arch Gen Psychiatry 2006;63(3):332–9.

9. Cipriani A, Zhou X, Del Giovane C, et al. Comparative efficacy and tolerability of antidepressants for major depressive disorder in children and adolescents: a network meta-analysis. Lancet 2016;388(10047):881–90.

10. Goldner EM, Jones W, Fang ML. Access to and waiting time for psychiatrist services in a Canadian urban area: a study in real time. Can J Psychiatry 2011;56(8): 474–80.

11. Donaldson AE, Gordon MS, Melvin GA, et al. Addressing the needs of adolescents with treatment resistant depressive disorders: a systematic review of rTMS. Brain Stimul 2014;7(1):7–12.

12. Wall CA, Croarkin PE, Maroney-Smith MJ, et al. Magnetic resonance imaging-guided, open-label, high-frequency repetitive transcranial magnetic stimulation for adolescents with major depressive disorder. J Child Adolesc Psychopharmacol 2016;26(7):582–9.

13. McClintock SM, Reti IM, Carpenter LL, et al. Consensus recommendations for the clinical application of repetitive transcranial magnetic stimulation (rTMS) in the treatment of depression. J Clin Psychiatry 2018;79(1) [pii:16cs10905].

14. O'Reardon JP, Solvason HB, Janicak PG, et al. Efficacy and safety of transcranial magnetic stimulation in the acute treatment of major depression: a multisite randomized controlled trial. Biol Psychiatry 2007;62(11):1208–16.

15. George MS, Lisanby SH, Avery D, et al. Daily left prefrontal transcranial magnetic stimulation therapy for major depressive disorder: a sham-controlled randomized trial. Arch Gen Psychiatry 2010;67(5):507–16.

16. Croarkin PE, Rotenberg A. Pediatric neuromodulation comes of age. J Child Adolesc Psychopharmacol 2016;26(7):578–81.

17. Lisanby SH. Noninvasive brain stimulation for depression - The devil is in the dosing. N Engl J Med 2017;376(26):2593–4.

18. Grabb MC, Gobburu JVS. Challenges in developing drugs for pediatric CNS disorders: a focus on psychopharmacology. Prog Neurobiol 2017;152:38–57.

19. Lefaucheur JP, Andre-Obadia N, Antal A, et al. Evidence-based guidelines on the therapeutic use of repetitive transcranial magnetic stimulation (rTMS). Clin Neurophysiol 2014;125(11):2150–206.

20. Brunoni AR, Chaimani A, Moffa AH, et al. Repetitive transcranial magnetic stimulation for the acute treatment of major depressive episodes: a systematic review with network meta-analysis. JAMA Psychiatry 2017;74(2):143–52.

21. Li CT, Chen MH, Juan CH, et al. Efficacy of prefrontal theta-burst stimulation in refractory depression: a randomized sham-controlled study. Brain 2014;137(Pt 7):2088–98.

22. Chung SW, Hoy KE, Fitzgerald PB. Theta-burst stimulation: a new form of TMS treatment for depression? Depress Anxiety 2015;32(3):182–92.

23. Hunter AM, Cook IA, Greenwald SD, et al. The antidepressant treatment response index and treatment outcomes in a placebo-controlled trial of fluoxetine. J Clin Neurophysiol 2011;28(5):478–82.

24. Blumberger DM, Vila-Rodriguez F, Thorpe KE, et al. Effectiveness of theta burst versus high-frequency repetitive transcranial magnetic stimulation in patients

with depression (THREE-D): a randomised non-inferiority trial. Lancet 2018; 391(10131):1683–92.

25. Walter G, Tormos JM, Israel JA, et al. Transcranial magnetic stimulation in young persons: a review of known cases. J Child Adolesc Psychopharmacol 2001;11(1): 69–75.

26. Loo C, McFarquhar T, Walter G. Transcranial magnetic stimulation in adolescent depression. Australas Psychiatry 2006;14(1):81–5.

27. Bloch Y, Grisaru N, Harel EV, et al. Repetitive transcranial magnetic stimulation in the treatment of depression in adolescents: an open-label study. J ECT 2008; 24(2):156–9.

28. Wall CA, Croarkin PE, Sim LA, et al. Adjunctive use of repetitive transcranial magnetic stimulation in depressed adolescents: a prospective, open pilot study. J Clin Psychiatry 2011;72(9):1263–9.

29. Mayer G, Aviram S, Walter G, et al. Long-term follow-up of adolescents with resistant depression treated with repetitive transcranial magnetic stimulation. J ECT 2012;28(2):84–6.

30. Le K, Liu L, Sun M, et al. Transcranial magnetic stimulation at 1 Hertz improves clinical symptoms in children with Tourette syndrome for at least 6 months. J Clin Neurosci 2013;20(2):257–62.

31. Yang XR, Kirton A, Wilkes TC, et al. Glutamate alterations associated with transcranial magnetic stimulation in youth depression: a case series. J ECT 2014; 30(3):242–7.

32. Farzan F, Dhami P, Atluri S, et al. Effiacy and biological targets of theta burst stimulation in treatment of youth depression. 2nd Annual International Brain Stimulation Conference. Barcelona, Spain, March 5–8, 2017.

33. MacMaster F, Croarkin P, Wilkes TC, et al. Open trial of repetitive transcranial magnetic stimulation in youth with treatment-resistant major depression. Biological Phychiatry 2018;83(9):S389–90.

34. Walter G, Martin J, Kirkby K, et al. Transcranial magnetic stimulation: experience, knowledge and attitudes of recipients. Aust N Z J Psychiatry 2001;35(1):58–61.

35. Croarkin PE, Nakonezny PA, Wall CA, et al. Transcranial magnetic stimulation potentiates glutamatergic neurotransmission in depressed adolescents. Psychiatry Res 2016;247:25–33.

36. Krishnan C, Santos L, Peterson MD, et al. Safety of noninvasive brain stimulation in children and adolescents. Brain Stimul 2015;8(1):76–87.

37. Davis NJ. Transcranial stimulation of the developing brain: a plea for extreme caution. Front Hum Neurosci 2014;8:600.

38. Geddes L. Brain stimulation in children spurs hope - and concern. Nature 2015; 525(7570):436–7.

39. Rossi S, Hallett M, Rossini PM, et al. Safety, ethical considerations, and application guidelines for the use of transcranial magnetic stimulation in clinical practice and research. Clin Neurophysiol 2009;120(12):2008–39.

40. Perera T, George MS, Grammer G, et al. The clinical TMS society consensus review and treatment recommendations for TMS therapy for major depressive disorder. Brain Stimul 2016;9(3):336–46.

41. Wu CS, Liu HY, Tsai HJ, et al. Seizure risk associated with antidepressant treatment among patients with depressive disorders: a population-based case-crossover study. J Clin Psychiatry 2017;78(9):e1226–32.

42. Allen CH, Kluger BM, Buard I. Safety of transcranial magnetic stimulation in children: a systematic review of the literature. Pediatr Neurol 2017;68:3–17.

43. Chiramberro M, Lindberg N, Isometsa E, et al. Repetitive transcranial magnetic stimulation induced seizures in an adolescent patient with major depression: a case report. Brain Stimul 2013;6(5):830–1.
44. Hu SH, Wang SS, Zhang MM, et al. Repetitive transcranial magnetic stimulation-induced seizure of a patient with adolescent-onset depression: a case report and literature review. J Int Med Res 2011;39(5):2039–44.
45. Cullen KR, Jasberg S, Nelson B, et al. Seizure induced by deep transcranial magnetic stimulation in an adolescent with depression. J Child Adolesc Psychopharmacol 2016;26(7):637–41.
46. Therapy NA. Safety and effectiveness of NeuroStar® transcranial magnetic stimulation (TMS) Therapy in depressed adolescents. 2015. Available at: https://www.clinicaltrials.gov/ct2/show/NCT02586688. Accessed May 27, 2018.
47. Dubin MJ, Mao X, Banerjee S, et al. Elevated prefrontal cortex GABA in patients with major depressive disorder after TMS treatment measured with proton magnetic resonance spectroscopy. J Psychiatry Neurosci 2016;41(3):E37–45.
48. Croarkin PE. Biomarkers in repetitive transcranial magnetic stimulation (rTMS) for adolescent depression 2018. 2018. Available at: https://www.clinicaltrials.gov/ct2/show/NCT03363919. Accessed May 27, 2018.
49. Croarkin PE, Levinson AJ, Daskalakis ZJ. Evidence for GABAergic inhibitory deficits in major depressive disorder. Neurosci Biobehav Rev 2011;35(3):818–25.
50. Sanacora G, Treccani G, Popoli M. Towards a glutamate hypothesis of depression: an emerging frontier of neuropsychopharmacology for mood disorders. Neuropharmacology 2012;62(1):63–77.
51. Vaiva G, Thomas P, Ducrocq F, et al. Low posttrauma GABA plasma levels as a predictive factor in the development of acute posttraumatic stress disorder. Biol Psychiatry 2004;55(3):250–4.
52. Valle AC, Dionisio K, Pitskel NB, et al. Low and high frequency repetitive transcranial magnetic stimulation for the treatment of spasticity. Dev Med Child Neurol 2007;49(7):534–8.
53. Gabbay V, Mao X, Klein RG, et al. Anterior cingulate cortex gamma-aminobutyric acid in depressed adolescents: relationship to anhedonia. Arch Gen Psychiatry 2012;69(2):139–49.
54. Price JL, Drevets WC. Neurocircuitry of mood disorders. Neuropsychopharmacology 2010;35(1):192–216.
55. Croarkin PE, Nakonezny PA, Husain MM, et al. Evidence for increased glutamatergic cortical facilitation in children and adolescents with major depressive disorder. JAMA Psychiatry 2013;70(3):291–9.
56. Gabbay V, Johnson AR, Alonso CM, et al. Anhedonia, but not irritability, is associated with illness severity outcomes in adolescent major depression. J Child Adolesc Psychopharmacol 2015;25(3):194–200.
57. Zhang W, Rosenkranz JA. Effects of repeated stress on age-dependent GABAergic regulation of the lateral nucleus of the amygdala. Neuropsychopharmacology 2016;41(9):2309–23.
58. Gilad GM, Gilad VH, Wyatt RJ, et al. Region-selective stress-induced increase of glutamate uptake and release in rat forebrain. Brain Res 1990;525(2):335–8.
59. Lowy MT, Gault L, Yamamoto BK. Adrenalectomy attenuates stress-induced elevations in extracellular glutamate concentrations in the hippocampus. J Neurochem 1993;61(5):1957–60.
60. Fontella FU, Vendite DA, Tabajara AS, et al. Repeated restraint stress alters hippocampal glutamate uptake and release in the rat. Neurochem Res 2004;29(9):1703–9.

61. Ehrlich DE, Ryan SJ, Hazra R, et al. Postnatal maturation of GABAergic transmission in the rat basolateral amygdala. J Neurophysiol 2013;110(4):926–41.
62. Krnjevic K, Randic M, Straughan DW. Nature of a cortical inhibitory process. J Physiol 1966;184(1):49–77.
63. Krnjevic K, Randic M, Straughan DW. An inhibitory process in the cerebral cortex. J Physiol 1966;184(1):16–48.
64. Ziemann U. Pharmacology of TMS. Suppl Clin Neurophysiol 2003;56:226–31.
65. Ziemann U, Reis J, Schwenkreis P, et al. TMS and drugs revisited 2014. Clin Neurophysiol 2015;126(10):1847–68.
66. Lewis CP, Nakonezny PA, Blacker CJ, et al. Cortical inhibitory markers of lifetime suicidal behavior in depressed adolescents. Neuropsychopharmacology 2018; 43(9):1822–31.
67. Lewis CP, Nakonezny PA, Ameis SH, et al. Cortical inhibitory and excitatory correlates of depression severity in children and adolescents. J Affect Disord 2016; 190:566–75.
68. Dyke K, Pepes SE, Chen C, et al. Comparing GABA-dependent physiological measures of inhibition with proton magnetic resonance spectroscopy measurement of GABA using ultra-high-field MRI. Neuroimage 2017;152:360–70.
69. Lewis CP, Port JD, Frye MA, et al. An exploratory study of spectroscopic glutamatergic correlates of cortical excitability in depressed adolescents. Front Neural Circuits 2016;10:98.
70. Beam W, Borckardt JJ, Reeves ST, et al. An efficient and accurate new method for locating the F3 position for prefrontal TMS applications. Brain Stimul 2009;2(1): 50–4.
71. Mir-Moghtadaei A, Caballero R, Fried P, et al. Concordance between BeamF3 and MRI-neuronavigated target sites for repetitive transcranial magnetic stimulation of the left dorsolateral prefrontal cortex. Brain Stimul 2015;8(5):965–73.
72. Poznanski EO, Grossman JA, Buchsbaum Y, et al. Preliminary studies of the reliability and validity of the children's depression rating scale. J Am Acad Child Psychiatry 1984;23(2):191–7.

Transcranial Magnetic Stimulation in Conditions Other than Major Depressive Disorder

Jonathan Essary Becker, DO, MS*, Elizabeth K.B. Shultz, DO, Christopher Todd Maley, MD

KEYWORDS

- Transcranial magnetic stimulation • Major depressive disorder
- Obsessive compulsive disorder • Autism spectrum disorder • Schizophrenia
- Attention-deficit/hyperactivity disorder

KEY POINTS

- Transcranial magnetic stimulation (TMS) is a treatment approved by the Food and Drug Administration for major depressive disorder (MDD). TMS is a neuromodulation technique that works by creating a focal magnetic field that induces a small electric current. Compared with other neuromodulation techniques (electroconvulsive therapy, deep brain stimulation, vagus nerve stimulation), TMS is a noninvasive treatment modality that is generally well-tolerated.
- Because of the success of TMS in treating depression, there has been interest in applications for other neuropsychiatric diseases, including schizophrenia, obsessive compulsive disorder, posttraumatic stress disorder, attention-deficit/hyperactivity disorder, substance use disorders, and autism spectrum disorders.
- The purpose of this article was to review potential uses for TMS for children and adolescents in conditions other than MDD.

INTRODUCTION

Transcranial magnetic stimulation (TMS) is a treatment approved by the Food and Drug Administration (FDA) for major depressive disorder (MDD). The FDA cleared the first TMS machine, Neuronetics, in 2008 for patients with MDD who failed 1 adequate medication trial during the current episode. TMS is a neuromodulation technique that works by creating a focal magnetic field that induces a small electric

Department of Psychiatry and Behavioral Sciences, Vanderbilt University Medical Center, 1601 23rd Avenue South, Nashville, TN 37212, USA
* Corresponding author.
E-mail address: jonathan.e.becker@vanderbilt.edu

Child Adolesc Psychiatric Clin N Am 28 (2019) 45–52
https://doi.org/10.1016/j.chc.2018.08.001
1056-4993/19/© 2018 Elsevier Inc. All rights reserved.

childpsych.theclinics.com

current. To create a prescribed dose, the machine creates these currents using pulses of varying amounts of strength, frequency (defined in Hz), and interval rest period without stimulation. This is modified by the total amount of time the magnet is placed over a targeted brain region. By doing this, the magnetic field stimulus can alter the firing patterns of the brain regions located underneath the magnet. Because of the success of TMS in treating depression, there has been interest in applications for other neuropsychiatric diseases. The purpose of this article was to review potential uses for TMS for children and adolescents in conditions other than MDD.

To treat depression, the standard treatment protocol targets the left dorsolateral prefrontal cortex (DLPFC). The left DLPFC was chosen because brain imaging research demonstrated decreased activity of this area in patients with depression and an association of this area with the behavioral dysregulation seen in depression (decreased energy, sleep-wake cycle disruption, appetite changes).[1] The standard approach to this target uses a stimulus delivered at 120% above the patient motor threshold (strength), 10 pulses per second (10 Hz) for 4 seconds with a 26-second interval period.[2] During that time, the patient receives a total of 3000 pulses. The repetitive stimulation pattern in this dosing is defined as repetitive high-frequency (greater than 1 Hz) TMS (HF rTMS). The proposed mechanism of action is that HF rTMS increases neuronal firing in this region, thus increasing its activity to modulate the neural circuit.[3] Alternatively, low-frequency rTMS (LF rTMS) applies a stimulus pulse at 1 pulse per second (1 Hz), which decreases neuronal firing with resultant decreased regional brain activity.[4]

Compared with other neuromodulation techniques (electroconvulsive therapy, deep brain stimulation, vagus nerve stimulation), TMS is a noninvasive treatment modality that is generally well tolerated. The most serious potential side effect is seizure, although in a review of more than 10,000 treatments in adults, using the figure 8 coil most common in clinical practice, there were no reported seizures.[5] McClintock and colleagues[6] estimated the risk of rTMS-induced seizure in adults to be 1 in 30,000. The risk is higher for patients with risk factors for seizures, such as a history of traumatic brain injury and those receiving higher than recommended doses of rTMS. LF rTMS is believed to be less likely to induce a seizure and may be used as an alternative approach to HF rTMS for those at risk for seizures. Safety data in children and adolescents is more limited; however, thought to be similar to safety data in adults. Allen and colleagues[7] completed a meta-analysis of 42 safety studies using single-pulse or paired-pulse TMS involving 639 healthy subjects, 482 subjects with central nervous system disorders, and 89 subjects with epilepsy, as well as 23 repetitive TMS studies involving 230 central nervous systems and 24 children with epilepsy and 3 theta-burst stimulation (TBS) studies involving 90 healthy children, 40 children with central nervous system disorder, and no epileptic children. Overall, they concluded that adverse events were rare in children and adolescents and typically mild, such as headache or tingling sensations. They found a total of 3 incidences of seizures and 1 incidence of induced hypomania with rTMS, which is similar to the incidence of these events in adults.

Given the ability of TMS to modulate neuronal firing in both excitatory and inhibitory ways in a clinically safe manner, interest has grown in TMS as a useful tool for a treatment of a variety of neuropsychiatric illnesses. Interest has expanded into other disorders, including schizophrenia, obsessive compulsive disorder (OCD), posttraumatic stress disorder (PTSD), attention-deficit/hyperactivity disorder (ADHD), substance use disorders, and autism spectrum disorders (ASDs).

OBSESSIVE COMPULSIVE DISORDER

In comparison with some other psychiatric illnesses, there is a better understanding of the neural cortico-striatal-thalamic-cortical circuits involved in the pathogenesis of OCD. Consequently, clinical interest has developed in using rTMS for refractory OCD. The supplementary motor area (SMA) and orbitofrontal cortex (OFC) exhibit hyperexcitability in OCD, which has led to the application of LF rTMS to reverse this hyperactivity.[8] Berlim and colleagues[9] conducted a meta-analysis of rTMS for OCD in adults including 10 studies and 282 subjects. They found that LF rTMS over the SMA or OFC demonstrated promising results and reported a 35% response rate for active versus 13% response rate for sham treatment, resulting in a number needed to treat of 5. Treatment of the left dorsolateral prefrontal cortex with high frequency showed no effect. These results were similar to the review by Bais and colleagues[10] of neuromodulation in OCD. One key concern raised in this review, though, was that the effect may not sustain after rTMS is stopped. Despite the promising initial results of studies included in these 2 reviews, a more recent randomized, double-blind, sham-controlled, trial of LF rTMS over the SMA failed to show a significant difference between the 2 groups.[11] Of note, this study only looked at treatment using LF rTMS over the SMA. Trevizol and colleagues[12] conducted another meta-analysis that included 15 studies. They found that rTMS was superior to sham TMS with no difference between high frequency and low frequency or site of stimulation.

The only study on rTMS for OCD in children and adolescents was a small study conducted by Pedapati and colleagues.[13] They used active and sham rTMS to compare functional MRI changes after a single rTMS treatment using 1800 pulses at 1-Hz frequency over the right dorsolateral prefrontal cortex. They found no difference in neural activity before and after treatment between the 2 groups. Taking all of this into consideration, the long-term usefulness and ideal treatment protocol for rTMS in pediatric OCD remain to be determined.

AUTISM SPECTRUM DISORDER

One of the other emerging areas of interest for the use of TMS is with regard to ASD, both for assessment and for treatment. Historically, TMS investigations in ASD have examined cortical plasticity, inhibition, and excitation as an assessment tool in learning about brain function in ASD. In more recent years, there have been case reports and studies examining the role of TMS in managing common symptoms of ASD as well as co-occurring depression.

In 2014, a case report highlighted the use of TMS in a 15-year-old male patient with both ASD and MDD.[14] The autism symptoms endorsed pretreatment included "limitations in social interactions, difficulties coping with change, stereotypic movements and behaviors, and limited and stereotypical language use"; depressive symptoms endorsed included "lack of motivation, decreased participation in activities, isolation, and crying spells," as well as "irritability and long-standing extreme sensitivity to negative emotion expressed by his twin brother." He received LF TMS initially over the right DLPFC to target mood symptoms. A series of 10 treatments at 90% of the resting motor threshold (RMT) were administered with pulses of 10 seconds on and 10 to 30 seconds off. Initially, he received 150 pulses per second (PPS) and then up to 300 PPS during the second week. He experienced improvement in mood symptoms by the end of the 10 sessions. Additionally, he received a course of LF TMS over the left DLPFC to target autism symptoms. The course included 10 sessions at 90% RMT with 300 PPS titrated to 600 PPS the second week. He tolerated the treatment with minimal side effects, and he experienced improvement in the aforementioned autism symptoms.

A more recent 2016 case-control study examined the effects of TMS via intermittent TBS (iTBS) on motor cortex plasticity (M1) in adolescents with ASD.[15] Their hypothesis purports that "the motor system develops differently in ASD"; thus, they used "repetitive TMS to probe the M1 using a protocol (iTBS) protocol" that they had used before to elicit cortical excitability in youth. According to the investigators, TBS is a type of TMS that specifically targets M1 to produce rather profound plasticity effects that can last approximately 10 to 90 minutes after administration. They hypothesized that via the protocol they would be able to identify a potential measure to "modulate these networks" (involved in M1 output) and "track treatment response," as they anticipated that the ASD participants would have increased excitability versus the case-control group. The protocol consisted of iTBS sessions with 300 PPS at 70% RMT for a total of 30 minutes. Their findings supported their hypothesis and suggest that there is increased cortical excitability youth with ASD. These findings may inspire investigation into uses of TBS for further assessment or perhaps treatment.

In 2014, Sokhadze and colleagues[16] published the results of a study examining the use of rTMS and neurofeedback (NFB) to modulate quantitative electroencephalogram (EEG) gamma waves by engaging the participants in a reaction time task as a type of sensory stimulation. Study groups included a "Waitlist" group that received no intervention and an rTMS plus NFB group. Participants who received rTMS + NFB had weekly sessions for 18 weeks with 6 treatments over the left DLPFC, 6 treatments over the right DLPFC, and the final 6 treatments were bilateral. Stimulation was administered at 90% of the motor threshold. NFB was implemented immediately after rTMS sessions in the form of 20-minute sessions following a "Focus/Neureka!" protocol using EEG. Social and behavioral functioning were evaluated before and after treatment, as well. The findings suggest that "rTMS-NFB treatment may have facilitated attention and target discrimination by improving conflict resolutions during processing task-relevant and task-irrelevant stimuli." Additionally, the results imply that rTMS can help improve the ratio of excitability to inhibitory responses, as well as that NFB may increase gamma activity. Participants were better able to reduce the number of errors or overreactive responses during assessments. Furthermore, they also had reductions in repetitive and stereotypic actions, as well as hyperactivity and lethargy ratings at the end of the study.

Upcoming future directions of TMS research include a clinical trial outlined by Ameis and colleagues[17] to examine the effect of TMS on executive function in adolescents and young adults with ASD. In this double-blind, sham-controlled, randomized controlled study protocol, participants will receive TMS applied bilaterally (first left or right and then the other side at each session) to DLPFC 5 d/wk for 4 weeks. Active treatment would occur at 90% RMT with 25 stimulation trains at 30 stimuli a piece and a break of 30 seconds between each train. Assessments before and after treatment include executive function testing as well as high-resolution MRI of the brain. Cognitive measures will be reassessed also at 1 month, 6 months, and 1 year after completion of the treatment. This study is currently ongoing at time of publication and does not yet have published results available.

SCHIZOPHRENIA

Studies examining the utility of TMS for schizophrenia in adults have generally focused on treatment of positive symptoms (primarily auditory hallucinations) using LF (1 Hz) TMS targeting the left temporoparietal cortex.[18] Studies examining the treatment of negative symptoms (avolition, apathy, cognitive dulling) have focused on higher-frequency TMS applied to the dorsolateral prefrontal cortex.[19] Overall, results have been inconsistent, and recent larger reviews have not found sufficient evidence to recommend the routine use of TMS for schizophrenia in adults.[20,21]

The literature regarding the use of TMS for the treatment of children and adolescents with schizophrenia is admittedly limited, although there are a number of case reports and small cohort studies suggesting that TMS may be of benefit.[22] In 2007, Jardri and colleagues[23] described a case in which an 11-year-old boy with very early onset schizophrenia was treated with LF (1 Hz) TMS over the left temporoparietal cortex. Symptoms before treatment included auditory hallucinations, alien control phenomena, and agitation. The patient received 10 sessions and experienced significant improvement in his auditory hallucinations (measured by the Auditory Hallucination Rating Scale) as well as improvement in his adaptive functioning as measured by the Children's Global Assessment Scale.

Jardri's group[24] later examined a cohort of adolescents who had been diagnosed with childhood-onset schizophrenia. In this series, 10 individuals (7 boys, 3 girls) with antipsychotic-resistant auditory hallucinations received LF (1 Hz) TMS applied to the left temporoparietal junction. Patients were treated with a stable antipsychotic regimen before receiving TMS. During the study, each patient received 10 total treatments (twice daily for 5 days). Overall, the group experienced significant decreases in auditory hallucinations (again, measured by the Auditory Hallucinations Rating Scale) as well as significant improvement in Global Assessment of Functioning scores. Improvements in both domains were sustained over the 1-month follow-up period. Treatment was generally well tolerated with only mild scalp discomfort reported as a side effect.[24]

In a 2006 study, Fitzgerald and colleagues[25] described treatment of an 18-year-old who had been diagnosed with childhood-onset schizophrenia at the age of 9. Before TMS, she had been treated with an adequate dose of clozapine but continued to experience significant, impairing auditory hallucinations. She was treated with 10 sessions of 1-Hz stimulation to the left temporoparietal cortex and experienced significant improvement in her hallucinations, which lasted for approximately 5 months (her clozapine dose remained unchanged over that time). She later received an additional 10 treatments and experienced a near-total resolution of hallucinations that lasted for another 3 months. She received a third course of TMS, this time consisting of 15 treatments and experienced similar improvement in hallucinations that persisted for 4 months posttreatment.

In a 2001 review, Walter and colleagues[26] described three 18-year-old male patients diagnosed with schizophrenia who received TMS. Each patient received 10 treatments over 2 weeks consisting of 20-Hz stimulation to the right frontal cortex. For one patient, rating scales scores were not available, but the review indicates that the patient and parents subjectively reported a decrease in hallucinatory experiences and in agitation. For the remaining 2 patients, improvement in both total and composite scores in the SANS (Schedule for the Assessment of Negative Symptoms) and SAPS (Schedule for the Assessment of Positive Symptoms) were observed.

ATTENTION-DEFICIT/HYPERACTIVITY DISORDER

ADHD is one of the most commonly treated psychiatric conditions. Although effective, treatment with stimulants does carry some concern for cardiovascular side effects, raising interest in alternative treatment methods. As discussed previously, TMS can be used to either increase or inhibit neuronal activity. Additionally, some research has demonstrated that TMS can affect the dopamine system in ways similar to D-amphetamine.[27–29] With this, and the established safety profile of TMS, there is the possibility for TMS to be a safe and effective treatment modality for ADHD. A small pilot study was first conducted by Bloch and colleagues[27] in 2010 in which they conducted a randomized controlled study with 13 adult patients with ADHD. HF (20-Hz) rTMS was used over the right dorsolateral prefrontal cortex at 100% motor threshold intensity. They found that rTMS was found to improve attention as measured by the Positive and Negative Affect Schedule attention score. Overall, they concluded that this effect was "modest with questionable clinical relevance."

The only randomized controlled trial in adolescents was conducted by Weaver and colleagues[30] in 2012. They randomized 9 adolescents and young adults between the ages of 14 and 21 to receive either active or sham HF rTMS over the right dorsolateral prefrontal cortex. Subjects received a 10-session course of TMS over 2 weeks, then there was a crossover phase. Although they found no statistically significant difference between active and sham treatment, they noted that subjects receiving active TMS in phase 2 began to show improvement over the sham group. They interpreted their findings in this small study to be encouraging for the potential efficacy of rTMS in the treatment of ADHD.

SUMMARY

At present, TMS appears to be a well-tolerated and safe treatment for children and adolescents, as it is with adults. There are many potential therapeutic uses for TMS, but further research is needed to determine the efficacy and to more clearly define the neural targets and stimulus dosing protocols for each condition. There are other potential neuropsychiatric illnesses for which TMS could prove to be an effective treatment not included in this review, such as eating disorders, migraine headaches, anxiety disorders, and PTSD.

In our clinical experience treating major depressive disorder, rTMS has been a successful and well-tolerated treatment for many patients who have suffered for years with refractory depression. The treatment has also been helpful in minimizing polypharmacy that often accompanies refractory depression and serves as an alternative, yet evidence-based, approach to treating patients who have struggled with medication side effects. Moving toward the future, we need to continue to build on the current evidence to develop clearly defined, standardized protocols for different neuropsychiatric conditions. Additionally, with the rapid pace at which uses for rTMS are expanding, clinicians can have a hard time keeping up with some of the newer protocols. Increased participation in national organizations, such as the Clinical TMS Society, can help train TMS providers in the most up-to-date information for clinical applications.

REFERENCES

1. Mayberg HS. Modulating dysfunctional limbic-cortical circuits in depression: towards development of brain-based algorithms for diagnosis and optimised treatment. Br Med Bull 2003;65:193–207.
2. George MS, Lisanby SH, Avery D, et al. Daily left prefrontal transcranial magnetic stimulation therapy for major depressive disorder a sham-controlled randomized trial. Arch Gen Psychiatry 2010;67(5):507–16.
3. Janicak PG, Dokucu ME. Transcranial magnetic stimulation for the treatment of major depression. Neuropsychiatr Dis Treat 2015;11:1549–60.
4. Speer AM, Kimbrell TA, Wassermann EM, et al. Opposite effects of high and low frequency rTMS on regional brain activity in depressed patients. Biol Psychiatry 2000;48(12):1133–41.

5. Janicak PG, O'Reardon JP, Sampson SM, et al. Transcranial magnetic stimulation in the treatment of major depressive disorder: a comprehensive summary of safety experience from acute exposure, extended exposure, and during reintroduction treatment. J Clin Psychiatry 2008;69(2):222–32.

6. McClintock SM, Reti IM, Carpenter LL, et al. Consensus recommendations for the clinical application of repetitive transcranial magnetic stimulation (rTMS) in the treatment of depression. J Clin Psychiatry 2018;79(1). https://doi.org/10.4088/JCP.16cs10905.

7. Allen CS, Kluger BM, Buard I. Safety of transcranial magnetic stimulation in children: a systematic review of the literature. Pediatr Neurol 2017;68:3–17.

8. Ahmari SE, Dougherty DD. Dissecting OCD circuits: from animal models to targeted treatments. Depress Anxiety 2015;32(8):550–62.

9. Berlim MT, Neufeld NH, Van den Eynde F. Repetitive transcranial magnetic stimulation (rTMS) for obsessive-compulsive disorder (OCD): an exploratory meta-analysis of randomized and sham-controlled trials. J Psychiatr Res 2013;47(8):999–1006.

10. Bais M, Figee M, Denys D. Neuromodulation in obsessive-compulsive disorder. Psychiatr Clin North Am 2014;37(3):393–413.

11. Pelissolo A, Harika-Germaneau G, Rachid F, et al. Repetitive transcranial magnetic stimulation to supplementary motor area in refractory obsessive-compulsive disorder treatment: a sham-controlled trial. Int J Neuropsychopharmacol 2016. https://doi.org/10.1093/ijnp/pyw025.

12. Trevizol AP, Shiozawa P, Cook IA, et al. Transcranial magnetic stimulation for obsessive-compulsive disorder: an updated systematic review and meta-analysis. J ECT 2016;32(4):262–6.

13. Pedapati E, Di Francesco M, Wu S, et al. Neural correlates associated with symptom provocation in pediatric obsessive compulsive disorder after a single session of sham-controlled repetitive transcranial magnetic stimulation. Psychiatry Res 2015;233(3):466–73.

14. Cristancho P, Akkineni K, Constantino JN, et al. Transcranial magnetic stimulation (TMS) in a 15 year old patient with autism and co-morbid depression. J ECT 2014;30(4):e46–7.

15. Pedapati EV, Gilbert DL, Erickson CA, et al. Abnormal cortical plasticity in youth with autism spectrum disorder: a transcranial magnetic stimulation case–control pilot study. J Child Adolesc Psychopharmacol 2016;26(7):625–31.

16. Sokhadze EM, El-Baz AS, Tasman A, et al. Neuromodulation integrating rTMS and neurofeedback for the treatment of autism spectrum disorder: an exploratory study. Appl Psychophysiol Biofeedback 2014;39(0):237–57.

17. Ameis SH, Daskalakis ZJ, Blumberger DM, et al. Repetitive transcranial magnetic stimulation for the treatment of executive function deficits in autism spectrum disorder: clinical trial approach. J Child Adolesc Psychopharmacol 2017;27(5):413–21.

18. Hoffman RE, Hawkins KA, Gueorguieva R, et al. Transcranial magnetic stimulation of left temporoparietal cortex and medication-resistant auditory hallucinations. Arch Gen Psychiatry 2003;60(1):49–56.

19. Dlabac-de Lange J, Knegtering R, Aleman A. Repetitive transcranial magnetic stimulation for negative symptoms of schizophrenia: review and meta-analysis. J Clin Psychiatry 2010;71(4):411–8.

20. Nieuwdorp W, Koops S, Somers M, et al. Transcranial magnetic stimulation, transcranial direct current stimulation and electroconvulsive therapy for medication-resistant psychosis of schizophrenia. Curr Opin Psychiatry 2015;28:222–8.

21. Dougall N, Maayan N, Soares-Weiser K, et al. Transcranial magnetic stimulation (TMS) for schizophrenia. Cochrane Database Syst Rev 2015;(8):CD006081.
22. Croarkin PE, Wall CA, Lee J. Applications of transcranial magnetic stimulation (TMS) in child and adolescent psychiatry. Int Rev Psychiatry 2011;23(5):445–53.
23. Jardri R, Lucas B, Delevoye-Turrell Y, et al. An 11-year-old boy with drug-resistant schizophrenia treated with temporo-parietal rTMS. Mol Psychiatry 2007;12(4):320.
24. Jardri R, Bubrovszky M, Demeulemeester M, et al. Repetitive transcranial magnetic stimulation to treat early-onset auditory hallucinations. J Am Acad Child Adolesc Psychiatry 2012;51(9):947–9.
25. Fitzgerald PB, Benitez J, Daskalakis JZ, et al. The treatment of recurring auditory hallucinations in schizophrenia with rTMS. World J Biol Psychiatry 2006;7(2):119–22.
26. Walter G, Tormos JM, Israel JA, et al. Transcranial magnetic stimulation in young persons: a review of known cases. J Child Adolesc Psychopharmacol 2001;11(1):69–75.
27. Bloch Y, Harel EV, Aviram S, et al. Positive effects of repetitive transcranial magnetic stimulation on attention in ADHD subjects: a randomized controlled pilot study. World J Biol Psychiatry 2010;11:755–8.
28. Strafekka AP, Paus T, Barrett J, et al. Repetitive transcranial magnetic stimulation of the human prefrontal cortex induces dopamine release in the caudate nucleus. J Neurosci 2001;21:RC157.
29. Pogarell O, Koch W, Popperi G, et al. Acute prefrontal rTMS increased striatal dopamine to a similar degree as D-amphetamine. Psychiatry Res 2007;156:251–5.
30. Weaver L, Rostain AL, Mace W, et al. Transcranial Magnetic Stimulation (TMS) in the treatment of attention deficit/hyperactivity disorder in adolescents and young adults: a pilot study. J ECT 2012;28(2):98–103.

Transcranial Direct Current Stimulation

Mechanisms and Psychiatric Applications

Daniel L. Kenney-Jung, MD[a], Caren J. Blacker, BMBCh, MA[b],
Deniz Doruk Camsari, MD[b], Jonathan C. Lee, MD, MSc[c,d],
Charles P. Lewis, MD[b,*]

KEYWORDS

- Transcranial direct current stimulation • Neuromodulation
- Noninvasive brain stimulation • Mechanisms • Applications

KEY POINTS

- Transcranial direct current stimulation (tDCS) is an emerging noninvasive brain stimulation modality involving weak electric current applied to the scalp.
- Mechanisms posited to underlie its effects include modification of cortical excitability, neural plasticity, and long-term potentiation/long-term depression processes.
- Clinical applications of tDCS have been studied increasingly in adults, particularly in mood disorders, and suggest antidepressant benefits.
- tDCS has been well tolerated in studies to date, with generally mild adverse effects.
- Future research focusing on how tDCS interacts with cognitive and behavioral processes may help maximize its therapeutic potential.

INTRODUCTION

Despite the prominence of medications in the treatment of psychiatric disorders, interest in alternative neurobiological treatments is growing. Noninvasive brain stimulation (NIBS) techniques target the brain directly, offering a rational approach for modulating network dysfunction in psychiatric disorders while limiting systemic effects.

Disclosures: C.J. Blacker, D. Doruk Camsari, and C.P. Lewis receive research support from the Mayo Clinic Foundation Departmental Small Grant Program. C.P. Lewis is a site investigator for multicenter studies funded by Neuronetics, Inc and NeoSync, Inc. D.L. Kenney-Jung and J. C. Lee have no financial disclosures.
[a] Department of Neurology, University of Minnesota, 420 Delaware Street SE, MMC 295, Minneapolis, MN 55455, USA; [b] Department of Psychiatry and Psychology, Division of Child and Adolescent Psychiatry, Mayo Clinic, 200 First Street SW, Rochester, MN 55905, USA; [c] Temerty Centre for Therapeutic Brain Intervention, Centre for Addiction and Mental Health, 1001 Queen Street W, Toronto, ON M6J 1H4, Canada; [d] Department of Psychiatry, Faculty of Medicine, University of Toronto, 250 College Street, Toronto, ON M5T 1R8, Canada
* Corresponding author.
E-mail address: Lewis.Charles@mayo.edu

Child Adolesc Psychiatric Clin N Am 28 (2019) 53–60
https://doi.org/10.1016/j.chc.2018.07.008
1056-4993/19/© 2018 Elsevier Inc. All rights reserved.

Transcranial direct current stimulation (tDCS) involves low-intensity electrical current applied to the scalp. Over the past 2 decades, tDCS has emerged as a method for modulating cortical excitability and enhancing cortical plasticity. Increasing evidence suggests clinical potential in adults with neuropsychiatric disorders, including epilepsy, stroke, and depression. In this article, the authors review the known neurobiological effects of tDCS and its adverse effects (AEs), summarize the emerging literature on tDCS for depression in adults, and discuss future directions in psychiatric tDCS research.

MECHANISMS OF TRANSCRANIAL DIRECT CURRENT STIMULATION

A tDCS device is straightforward: electrical stimulation is delivered at constant (direct) current through cathodal and anodal electrodes applied to the skin, driven by a small battery.[1,2] Typically, both anode and cathode are placed on the scalp,[3] although reference electrodes can be placed in an extracephalic location (eg, pectoral or deltoid muscles) to allow only cathodal or anodal stimulation of the targeted head region. Other montages involving multiple electrodes of one or both polarities also exist.[4] The current applied is generally weak, typically 1 to 2 mA. At any given current intensity, current density increases when electrode size decreases. Thus, if stimulation of one polarity is desired, increasing the size of the electrode of the opposite polarity emphasizes the stimulation of the desired polarity.

Although the precise physiologic mechanisms of tDCS remain to be elucidated, substantial in vitro and in vivo data exist. Generally, cathodal stimulation decreases neuronal excitability in the targeted area, whereas anodal stimulation increases it.[5] Anodal stimulation increases motor evoked potential (MEP) amplitudes,[5] and stimulation of visual cortex modulates phosphene thresholds.[6] These findings are complicated by research showing that intensity and length of stimulation impact the effects; in one study, cathodal stimulation at 1 mA induced inhibition, whereas 2 mA increased excitability of the MEP response.[7] In addition, cells of certain subpopulations may respond differently or be more sensitive to DC stimulation than others, due to location, connectivity, chemical subpopulation, or morphology.[8]

The orientation of neurons, dendrites, and axonal processes is important to the effects of electrical stimulation, because the direction of current flow impacts neuronal effects.[9–12] One advantage of tDCS, its noninvasive nature, complicates investigators' ability to understand the impact of transcranially applied current on underlying brain topography. Furthermore, how weak currents are propagated through scalp, skull, and the brain's complex tissue architecture remains an area of active research.

Modulation of the membrane potential at the neuronal soma has been posited as a potential mechanism of tDCS effects. Anodal stimulation can increase the spontaneous firing rate of neurons; similarly, cathodal stimulation can hyperpolarize neuronal membranes and diminish excitability. Notably, weak DC stimulation does not directly cause action potentials; rather, it increases or decreases membrane excitability by driving the membrane toward or away from its threshold potential.[13] Pharmacologic blockade of voltage-gated sodium channels can suppress short-term increases in excitability during tDCS, suggesting the role of membrane polarization in these effects.[9]

The therapeutic potential of tDCS hinges on the durability of poststimulation effects, yet these remain incompletely understood. Convergent findings suggest that long-term potentiation (LTP) and long-term depression (LTD) mechanisms are central to tDCS's persistent effects.[14,15] Chemical blockade of the N-methyl-D-aspartate glutamatergic receptor, important in LTP and in neuroplasticity and learning, can abolish aftereffects of tDCS.[9,16] In addition, persistent poststimulation effects require protein synthesis[1] and brain-derived neuronal growth factor,[17] both necessary for LTP. Moreover, performance on some learning tasks (likely mediated by LTP) improves with tDCS.[18] Dopaminergic and serotonergic neurotransmission also may play a role; dopaminergic blockade attenuates tDCS's aftereffects,[19,20] whereas citalopram, a serotonin reuptake inhibitor, can augment them.[21] Other phenomena, including cell migration (electro-taxis),[13] altered levels of intracellular calcium,[16] and altered levels and localization of various membrane receptors, may contribute to tDCS's persistent effects.

ADULT TRANSCRANIAL DIRECT CURRENT STIMULATION STUDIES FOR DEPRESSION

Researchers have examined the efficacy and tolerability of tDCS extensively in adults, particularly in depression. Several large trials have compared tDCS with sham stimu-lation and pharmacologic treatments. One open-label crossover trial involving 3 phases (6-week acute treatment, crossover, and maintenance therapy for responders) compared tDCS to sertraline for major depressive disorder (MDD).[22,23] tDCS was su-perior to placebo during acute-phase treatment, and it had an additive effect when used concurrently with sertraline.[22] AEs were generally mild, with skin redness re-ported in active tDCS, and 7 participants experiencing mania or hypomania. Patients who received sham tDCS plus placebo were eligible for the crossover phase, and all responders from both acute phases were enrolled in the 6-month follow-up phase. Few AEs were reported during follow-up, and none experienced manic/hypomanic switch. Higher-than-expected dropout was observed, potentially related to the burden of traveling for treatments. Another study compared tDCS with escitalopram[24] and found significant improvement in depression severity with tDCS versus placebo, although tDCS did not demonstrate noninferiority to escitalopram. AEs were similar across all treatment groups, and 2 patients developed mania.

Several meta-analyses pooled data from open-label tDCS studies and randomized controlled trials (RCTs) for MDD. A limited number of RCTs have been conducted, result-ing in substantial overlap of data across meta-analyses. A meta-analysis of open-label trials and RCTs in a pooled population of 176 adults[25] found that active tDCS reduced depression severity more than sham, but was limited by small sample size. A similar re-view, which included one additional study for a population of 200 patients, divided RCTs into those using tDCS as adjunctive/combination therapy versus those using tDCS as monotherapy.[26] Meta-analysis of all RCTs found no difference in response or remission rates, but analysis of monotherapy trials found significantly higher response rates for active tDCS than sham. A later meta-analysis of 259 pooled patients[27] found that tDCS had significantly higher response and remission rates than sham, with significant decreases in depression scores. Brunoni and colleagues[28] analyzed individual patient data of 289 pooled patients, finding tDCS superior to sham in the treatment of MDD, with an effect size comparable to transcranial magnetic stimulation (TMS) and antide-pressant medications. These meta-analyses suggest accumulating evidence for thera-peutic efficacy in adult MDD. The improvement over time may be partly attributable to the inclusion of trials with larger numbers of participants as the field progresses.

ADVERSE EFFECTS

Studies to date indicate that tDCS is well tolerated overall, with low dropout rates that are comparable between active and sham groups.[26–28] Most AEs reported in adults have been mild, including headache, tingling, itching, burning sensations, and local discomfort.[25] Relatively few AEs related to tDCS have been reported under typical protocols (1–2 mA currents and 0.03–0.08 mA/cm^2 current densities over 20–30 mi-nutes).[29] According to one survey in 102 patients,[30] the most common AEs after tDCS were headache (11.8%), nausea (2.9%), and insomnia (0.98%).

A systematic review[31] examined AEs in 209 experimental tDCS studies in healthy volunteers and patients with various clinical conditions. The most common AEs were mild sensory effects: itching (39.3%), tingling (22.2%), headache (14.8%), burning sensations (8.7%), and discomfort (10.4%). No statistically significant difference in AE frequency was observed between control and experimental groups, although studies involving older patients, patients with clinical conditions, and higher current densities were statistically more likely to report AEs. Substantial between-study heterogeneity was found, and 44% of studies did not comment on AEs; only 8 studies systematically quantified AEs. The investigators recommended systematic collection of AE data in future tDCS trials. A subsequent prospective study found a statistically significant increase in the incidence of mild sensory AEs in those receiving active tDCS compared with the sham control group.[32]

Skin lesions resembling burns or contact dermatitis have been reported.[29] Although the current used in tDCS is low, smaller electrodes increase charge density by distributing current over a smaller area. In one study, skin lesioning was observed when tap water was used for electrode conductance, but resolved when replaced with saline.[25] To avoid skin lesions, electrodes should be placed only over intact skin, saline should be used for conductance, and patients should be encouraged to report concerns or discomfort promptly. Although the use of topical anesthetics at electrode sites during stimulation has been discussed,[33] there is concern that this could mask the development of skin lesions.

Some research protocols have used extracephalic electrode placements. Concern exists that directing current outside the head could have undesirable autonomic effects (eg, respiratory depression or cardiac effects). One early study reported a case of respiratory arrest and hand cramping with preserved consciousness during tDCS, which resolved with cessation of stimulation.[34] Recently, Vandermeeren and colleagues[35] evaluated autonomic function in 30 patients receiving tDCS with extracephalic electrodes. No changes in autonomic function were discerned, and no AEs were reported.

Mania/hypomania has been reported among patients receiving tDCS in trials for depression or bipolar disorder, although this has occurred in the context of underlying mood disorders and medications that could induce mania/hypomania.[22,29] Although tDCS could directly precipitate mania/hypomania, it also is possible that a synergistic or augmentative effect occurs when tDCS is used alongside pharmacologic antidepressants. The latter possibility must be entertained in light of increased poststimulation effects observed with concurrent tDCS and citalopram.[21]

With any neurostimulatory modality, seizure potential must be considered. Some investigators view a seizure disorder as a relative contraindication for tDCS. Data on the role of tDCS in seizure induction, however, are scant. One case report[36] described a patient with preexisting seizure disorder (infantile spasms) who underwent tDCS for spasticity. The patient had a seizure 4 hours after a tDCS session; however, this occurred in the context of a recently altered anticonvulsant regimen.[29,36] A pediatric trial of tDCS for focal epilepsy, using 1-mA cathodal stimulation over the putative seizure focus and extracephalic localization (contralateral shoulder) for the anode, reported no AEs, including seizures.[37] Likewise, in a trial of patients receiving tDCS for medically refractory epilepsy, no patients experienced an increase in seizures after therapy.[38]

FUTURE DIRECTIONS IN TRANSCRANIAL DIRECT CURRENT STIMULATION RESEARCH

Many studies to date have examined tDCS as monotherapy or in combination with psychotropic medications. Emerging work suggests the promise of tDCS coupled with cognitive and psychotherapeutic interventions. The ability of tDCS to impact cortical processes instrumental to plasticity and learning underlies its potential to enhance skill acquisition in cognitive and behavioral interventions. Theoretically, this suggests the appealing prospect that patients who have failed to benefit adequately from psychotherapy or skills training might experience an enhanced response to these interventions when stimulation is added. The portability of tDCS devices and tolerability profile permit integration into other interventions that require movement, cognitive activity, or social interaction. In this regard, tDCS has clear advantages over other NIBS techniques, such as repetitive TMS. However, unanswered questions about how tDCS interacts with concurrent tasks complicate the translation of this principle to practice. Neural networks activated during a task may impact the effects of tDCS, as motor and cognitive processes have shown distinct effects on excitability.[39] Stimulation effects on trained versus untrained tasks also appear to differ.[40] Other task-specific properties may influence the effect of tDCS on performance, including cognitive demand,[41] active versus passive movement,[42] and speed.[43] The sequence of stimulation also is likely to be significant: tDCS delivered before a motor training task increases excitability of the motor cortex,[44] yet this increased excitability can be eliminated by both cognitive and motor activity after stimulation.[45,46] Furthermore, the number of sessions (single versus repeated) of concurrent stimulation and cognitive tasks may have differing excitability effects on different cortical locations.[47] Despite the complexity of task-related contexts, several early studies have used tDCS in conjunction with cue-based tasks to reduce cravings in addiction,[48–50] and to enhance exercise programs[51] and speech therapy.[52] How tDCS impacts learning and task enhancement in the developing brain remains largely unexplored, and future studies will be required to establish how stimulation and concurrent interventions interact as neural networks undergo maturation.

In this article, the authors have focused on stimulation paradigms using bipolar electrode arrangements (single anode and single cathode), yet there are montages with a greater number of electrodes designed to focus the stimulation effect ("high-density" tDCS). Other lines of research are pursuing alternatives to the uniform direct current used in tDCS. Transcranial alternating current stimulation uses an alternating electrical waveform whose frequency can be modified, offering the intriguing possibility of using stimulation to synchronize endogenous oscillatory brain activity, disruptions of which may underline symptoms of psychiatric disorders.[53–56] Another modality, transcranial random noise stimulation, uses current whose frequency and intensity vary randomly, which may increase synchronization and amplify endogenous oscillations by reducing endogenous noise.[56] Approaches with more complex electrical waveforms may lead to more precise targeting of network pathologies responsible for clinical conditions, ultimately permitting individualized treatments based on individual patients' endogenous brain activity.

In summary, tDCS research is a young but rapidly developing field, with substantial promise as a research tool and clinical intervention. Early physiologic studies have identified its ability to induce short-term and potentially longer-term effects on neural excitability and learning processes. Overall, AEs are mild in comparison to pharmacologic and other neuromodulatory interventions, and its favorable tolerability profile is a significant advantage for future clinical uses of tDCS. Increasing evidence from the adult literature suggests antidepressant effects, although tDCS has yet to obtain regulatory approval for this indication. Further research is needed to clarify the durability of effects and how tDCS can be applied in conjunction with cognitive and behavioral treatments to result in maximum therapeutic potential.

REFERENCES

1. Reinhart RMG, Cosman JD, Fukuda K, et al. Using transcranial direct-current stimulation (tDCS) to understand cognitive processing. Atten Percept Psychophys 2017;79:3–23.
2. Utz KS, Dimova V, Oppenländer K, et al. Electrified minds: transcranial direct current stimulation (tDCS) and galvanic vestibular stimulation (GVS) as methods of non-invasive brain stimulation in neuropsychology—a review of current data and future implications. Neuropsychologia 2010;48:2789–810.
3. DaSilva AF, Volz MS, Bikson M, et al. Electrode positioning and montage in transcranial direct current stimulation. J Vis Exp 2011;51:e2744.
4. Faria P, Hallett M, Miranda PC. A finite element analysis of the effect of electrode area and inter-electrode distance on the spatial distribution of the current density in tDCS. J Neural Eng 2011;8:066017.
5. Cambiaghi M, Velikova S, Gonzalez-Rosa JJ, et al. Brain transcranial direct current stimulation modulates motor excitability in mice. Eur J Neurosci 2010;31:704–9.
6. Antal A, Nitsche MA, Paulus W. External modulation of visual perception in humans. Neuroreport 2001;12(16):3553–5.
7. Batsikadze G, Moliadze V, Paulus W, et al. Partially non-linear stimulation intensity-dependent effects of direct current stimulation on motor cortex excitability in humans. J Physiol 2013;591:1987–2000.
8. Roche N, Geiger M, Bussel B. Mechanisms underlying transcranial direct current stimulation in rehabilitation. Ann Phys Rehabil Med 2015;58:214–9.
9. Nitsche MA, Liebetanz D, Schlitterlau A, et al. GABAergic modulation of DC stimulation-induced motor cortex excitability shifts in humans. Eur J Neurosci 2004;19:2720–6.
10. Kabakov AY, Muller PA, Pascual-Leone A, et al. Contribution of axonal orientation to pathway-dependent modulation of excitatory transmission by direct current stimulation in isolated rat hippocampus. J Neurophysiol 2012;107:1881–9.
11. Radman T, Ramos RL, Brumberg JC, et al. Role of cortical cell type and morphology in subthreshold and suprathreshold uniform electric field stimulation in vitro. Brain Stimul 2009;2:215–28, 228.e1–3.
12. Purpura DP, McMurtry JG. Intracellular activities and evoked potential changes during polarization of motor cortex. J Neurophysiol 1965;28:166–85.
13. Pelletier SJ, Cicchetti F. Cellular and molecular mechanisms of action of transcranial direct current stimulation: evidence from in vitro and in vivo models. Int J Neuropsychopharmacol 2015;18(2): pyu047.
14. Nitsche MA, Müller-Dahlhaus F, Paulus W, et al. The pharmacology of neuroplasticity induced by non-invasive brain stimulation: building models for the clinical use of CNS active drugs. J Physiol 2012;590:4641–62.
15. Kronberg G, Bridi M, Abel T, et al. Direct current stimulation modulates LTP and LTD: activity dependence and dendritic effects. Brain Stimul 2017;10:51–8.
16. Liebetanz D, Nitsche MA, Tergau F, et al. Pharmacological approach to the mechanisms of transcranial DC-stimulation-induced after-effects of human motor cortex excitability. Brain 2002;125:2238–47.
17. Fritsch B, Reis J, Martinowich K, et al. Direct current stimulation promotes BDNF-dependent synaptic plasticity: potential implications for motor learning. Neuron 2010;66:198–204.
18. Nitsche MA, Schauenburg A, Lang N, et al. Facilitation of implicit motor learning by weak transcranial direct current stimulation of the primary motor cortex in the human. J Cogn Neurosci 2003;15:619–26.

19. Monte-Silva K, Ruge D, Teo JT, et al. D2 receptor block abolishes theta burst stimulation-induced neuroplasticity in the human motor cortex. Neuropsychopharmacology 2011;36:2097–102.
20. Nitsche MA, Lampe C, Antal A, et al. Dopaminergic modulation of long-lasting direct current-induced cortical excitability changes in the human motor cortex. Eur J Neurosci 2006;23:1651–7.
21. Nitsche MA, Kuo M-F, Karrasch R, et al. Serotonin affects transcranial direct current–induced neuroplasticity in humans. Biol Psychiatry 2009;66:503–8.
22. Brunoni AR, Valiengo L, Baccaro A, et al. The sertraline vs electrical current therapy for treating depression clinical study: results from a factorial, randomized, controlled trial. JAMA Psychiatry 2013;70(4):383–91.
23. Valiengo L, Benseñor IM, Goulart AC, et al. The Sertraline versus Electrical Current Therapy for Treating Depression Clinical Study (SELECT-TDCS): results of the crossover and follow-up phases. Depress Anxiety 2013;30(7):646–53.
24. Brunoni AR, Moffa AH, Sampaio-Júnior B, et al. Trial of electrical direct-current therapy versus escitalopram for depression. N Engl J Med 2017;376(26): 2523–33.
25. Kalu UG, Sexton CE, Loo CK, et al. Transcranial direct current stimulation in the treatment of major depression: a meta-analysis. Psychol Med 2012;42(9):1791–800.
26. Berlim MT, Van den Eynde F, Daskalakis ZJ. Clinical utility of transcranial direct current stimulation (tDCS) for treating major depression: a systematic review and meta-analysis of randomized, double-blind and sham-controlled trials. J Psychiatr Res 2013;47(1):1–7.
27. Shiozawa P, Fregni F, Benseñor IM, et al. Transcranial direct current stimulation for major depression: an updated systematic review and meta-analysis. Int J Neuropsychopharmacol 2014;17(9):1443–52.
28. Brunoni AR, Moffa AH, Fregni F, et al. Transcranial direct current stimulation for acute major depressive episodes: meta-analysis of individual patient data. Br J Psychiatry 2016;208(6):522–31.
29. Matsumoto H, Ugawa Y. Adverse events of tDCS and tACS: a review. Clin Neurophysiol Pract 2017;2:19–25.
30. Poreisz C, Boros K, Antal A, et al. Safety aspects of transcranial direct current stimulation concerning healthy subjects and patients. Brain Res Bull 2007;72:208–14.
31. Brunoni AR, Amadera J, Berbel B, et al. A systematic review on reporting and assessment of adverse effects associated with transcranial direct current stimulation. Int J Neuropsychopharmacol 2011;14(8):1133–45.
32. Kessler SK, Turkeltaub PE, Benson JG, et al. Differences in the experience of active and sham transcranial direct current stimulation. Brain Stimul 2012;5:155–62.
33. McFadden JL, Borckardt JJ, George MS, et al. Reducing procedural pain and discomfort associated with transcranial direct current stimulation. Brain Stimul 2011;4:38–42.
34. Lippold OCJ, Redfearn JWT. Mental changes resulting from the passage of small direct currents through the human brain. Br J Psychiatry 1964;110:768–72.
35. Vandermeeren Y, Jamart J, Ossemann M. Effect of tDCS with an extracephalic reference electrode on cardio-respiratory and autonomic functions. BMC Neurosci 2010;11:38.
36. Ekici B. Transcranial direct current stimulation–induced seizure: analysis of a case. Clin EEG Neurosci 2015;46:169.
37. Auvichayapat N, Rotenberg A, Gersner R, et al. Transcranial direct current stimulation for treatment of refractory childhood focal epilepsy. Brain Stimul 2013;6: 696–700.

38. Fregni F, Thome-Souza S, Nitsche MA, et al. A controlled clinical trial of cathodal DC polarization in patients with refractory epilepsy. Epilepsia 2006;47:335–42.

39. Antal A, Terney D, Poreisz C, et al. Towards unravelling task-related modulations of neuroplastic changes induced in the human motor cortex. Eur J Neurosci 2007; 26(9):2687–91.

40. Elmasry J, Loo C, Martin D. A systematic review of transcranial electrical stimulation combined with cognitive training. Restor Neurol Neurosci 2015;33(3):263–78.

41. Gill J, Shah-Basak PP, Hamilton R. It's the thought that counts: examining the task-dependent effects of transcranial direct current stimulation on executive function. Brain Stimul 2015;8(2):253–9.

42. Miyaguchi S, Onishi H, Kojima S, et al. Corticomotor excitability induced by anodal transcranial direct current stimulation with and without non-exhaustive movement. Brain Res 2013;1529:83–91.

43. Bortoletto M, Pellicciari MC, Rodella C, et al. The interaction with task-induced activity is more important than polarization: a tDCS study. Brain Stimul 2015;8(2):269–76.

44. Cabral ME, Baltar A, Borba R, et al. Transcranial direct current stimulation: before, during, or after motor training? Neuroreport 2015;26(11):618–22.

45. Quartarone A, Morgante F, Bagnato S, et al. Long lasting effects of transcranial direct current stimulation on motor imagery. Neuroreport 2004;15(8):1287–91.

46. Thirugnanasambandam N, Sparing R, Dafotakis M, et al. Isometric contraction interferes with transcranial direct current stimulation (tDCS) induced plasticity: evidence of state-dependent neuromodulation in human motor cortex. Restor Neurol Neurosci 2011;29(5):311–20.

47. Conti CL, Moscon JA, Fregni F, et al. Cognitive related electrophysiological changes induced by non-invasive cortical electrical stimulation in crack-cocaine addiction. Int J Neuropsychopharmacol 2014;17(9):1465–75.

48. Boggio PS, Liguori P, Sultani N, et al. Cumulative priming effects of cortical stimulation on smoking cue-induced craving. Neurosci Lett 2009;463(1):82–6.

49. Fregni F, Liguori P, Fecteau S, et al. Cortical stimulation of the prefrontal cortex with transcranial direct current stimulation reduces cue-provoked smoking craving: a randomized, sham-controlled study. J Clin Psychiatry 2008;69(1):32–40.

50. Shahbabaie A, Golesorkhi M, Zamanian B, et al. State dependent effect of transcranial direct current stimulation (tDCS) on methamphetamine craving. Int J Neuropsychopharmacol 2014;17(10):1591–8.

51. Mendonca ME, Simis M, Grecco LC, et al. Transcranial direct current stimulation combined with aerobic exercise to optimize analgesic responses in fibromyalgia: a randomized placebo-controlled clinical trial. Front Hum Neurosci 2016;10:68.

52. Carvalho Lima VL, Collange Grecco LA, Marques VC, et al. Transcranial direct current stimulation combined with integrative speech therapy in a child with cerebral palsy: a case report. J Bodyw Mov Ther 2016;20(2):252–7.

53. Fröhlich F. Endogenous and exogenous electric fields as modifiers of brain activity: rational design of noninvasive brain stimulation with transcranial alternating current stimulation. Dialogues Clin Neurosci 2014;16(1):93–102.

54. Fröhlich F. Experiments and models of cortical oscillations as a target for noninvasive brain stimulation. Prog Brain Res 2015;222:41–73.

55. Fröhlich F, Sellers KK, Cordle AL. Targeting the neurophysiology of cognitive systems with transcranial alternating current stimulation. Expert Rev Neurother 2015; 15(2):145–67.

56. Antal A, Herrmann CS. Transcranial alternating current and random noise stimulation: possible mechanisms. Neural Plast 2016;2016:3616807.

Transcranial Direct Current Stimulation in Child and Adolescent Psychiatric Disorders

Jonathan C. Lee, MD, MSc[a,b], Daniel L. Kenney-Jung, MD[c],
Caren J. Blacker, BMBCh, MA[d], Deniz Doruk Camsari, MD[d],
Charles P. Lewis, MD[d,*]

KEYWORDS

- Transcranial direct current stimulation • Neuromodulation • Children • Adolescents
- Neurodevelopment

KEY POINTS

- Transcranial direct current stimulation (tDCS) affects cortical excitability via γ-aminobutyric acid (GABA)-ergic and glutamatergic systems, which undergo substantial developmental changes, along with cortical network and anatomic maturation.
- Research in youth has focused predominantly on autism spectrum disorder, attention-deficit hyperactivity disorder, and neurodevelopmental disorders.
- Preliminary evidence in children and adolescents suggests safety and tolerability across broad diagnostic groups; definitive efficacy data, however, are lacking.
- Larger, longitudinal studies examining how tDCS affects brain development are essential for developing safe, effective tDCS interventions for youth with psychiatric conditions.

INTRODUCTION

Transcranial direct current stimulation (tDCS) involves applying low-intensity electrical current to the scalp to modulate activity of the underlying cortex. Recently, researchers have studied tDCS in children and adolescents with psychotic,

Disclosures: C.J. Blacker, D. Doruk Camsari, and C.P. Lewis receive research support from the Mayo Clinic Foundation Departmental Small Grant Program. C.P. Lewis is a site investigator for multicenter studies funded by Neuronetics, Inc and NeoSync, Inc. J.C. Lee and D.L. Kenney-Jung have no financial disclosures.
[a] Temerty Centre for Therapeutic Brain Intervention, Centre for Addiction and Mental Health, 1001 Queen Street W, Toronto, ON M6J 1H4, Canada; [b] Department of Psychiatry, Faculty of Medicine, University of Toronto, 250 College Street, Toronto, ON M5T 1R8, Canada; [c] Department of Neurology, University of Minnesota, 420 Delaware Street SE, MMC 295, Minneapolis, MN 55455, USA; [d] Department of Psychiatry and Psychology, Division of Child and Adolescent Psychiatry, Mayo Clinic, 200 First Street SW, Rochester, MN 55905, USA
* Corresponding author.
E-mail address: Lewis.Charles@mayo.edu

Child Adolesc Psychiatric Clin N Am 28 (2019) 61–78
https://doi.org/10.1016/j.chc.2018.07.009
1056-4993/19/© 2018 Elsevier Inc. All rights reserved.

neurodevelopmental, and eating disorders. This nascent literature suggests both safety and potential therapeutic utility in these populations.[1–5] However, the use of neuromodulatory techniques in the young brain presents unique considerations, including effects on developing neural systems. This article discusses aspects of neural development pertinent to the use of tDCS in youth, reviews the pediatric literature examining safety and clinical effects, and discusses future applications in child and adolescent psychiatry.

CONSIDERATIONS IN PEDIATRIC APPLICATIONS OF TRANSCRANIAL DIRECT CURRENT STIMULATION

In light of putative effects on neuronal excitability and long-term potentiation and depression, tDCS studies in children and adolescents must consider the context of developing γ-aminobutyric acid (GABA) and glutamate systems. Animal and human studies show that GABAergic inhibitory tone increases gradually from the prenatal period to adulthood. This likely results from numerous mechanisms, including age-related changes in the relative expression of GABA and glutamate receptor subunits,[6] differential receptor expression across brain structures with age,[7] and developmental shifts in cotransporter expression that affect GABA receptor functioning.[8] $GABA_A$ receptors, the brain's main rapid-acting inhibitory receptors in adulthood, have a paradoxical excitatory effect in early development,[9] whereas postsynaptic inhibition (mediated by metabotropic $GABA_B$ receptors in the mature brain) is absent during early development.[9,10] Additionally, receptor–receptor interactions shift with development. In early life, N-methyl-D-aspartate (NMDA) glutamatergic receptors dominate excitatory neurotransmission, with α-amino-3-hydroxy-5-methyl-4-isoxazolepropionic acid (AMPA) receptors having little function, whereas AMPA-NMDA receptor synergism mediates fast excitatory transmission in the mature brain.[6,9] Other long-term maturational processes, including myelin deposition, pruning, and evolving connectivity, also affect cortical network excitability.[11] Although mechanistic studies of tDCS in youth are largely lacking, preliminary work highlights that caution should be exercised in assuming that the pediatric and adult brain respond similarly to tDCS. One pediatric study found that 1-mA cathodal tDCS had a paradoxical, excitatory effect on transcranial magnetic stimulation–measured cortical excitability.[12]

Computational modeling approaches can be used to estimate the effects of tDCS in children and adolescents by adapting adult tDCS data while accounting for differences between developing and mature brains. Various anatomic parameters change with age: thickness of the scalp and calvarium, scalp-to-brain distance, cerebrospinal fluid volume, and developmental changes in tissue architecture.[3,13] By incorporating these factors in computerized models, adult data can be extrapolated to predict the relative impact of current intensity, density, and distribution in youth undergoing tDCS. A greater proportion of current applied to the pediatric head is posited to reach the cortex,[3] resulting in peak electric fields approximately 1.5 to 2 times higher than in adults undergoing identical stimulation.[14,15] Nevertheless, many studies in children and adolescents have used adult parameters (eg, 2-mA currents) without adjustment. Despite higher predicted cortical penetration in children, modeling studies have concluded that 2-mA currents are at least an order of magnitude below intensities that produce tissue damage in rodent studies.[16,17] However, in the absence of studies directly evaluating the neural effects of tDCS in young human populations, some investigators have advocated more conservative dosing strategies.[1]

TRANSCRANIAL DIRECT CURRENT STIMULATION STUDIES IN CHILDREN AND ADOLESCENTS WITH PSYCHIATRIC DISORDERS

Despite few published studies to date, pediatric tDCS research is a worldwide endeavor, with studies originating from Brazil,[18,19] Egypt,[20] Germany,[21–25] Iran,[26,27] Italy,[28–32] Thailand,[33,34] and the United States.[35,36] Neurodevelopmental disorders, such as attention-deficit hyperactivity disorder (ADHD)[19,21–27] and autism spectrum disorder (ASD),[18,28,29,33,34,36] have been the conditions most extensively studied to date. Other studies have examined the effects of tDCS in children and adolescents with dyslexia and learning disorders,[30–32] childhood-onset schizophrenia (COS),[35] and eating disorders.[20] In a notable contrast to the adult literature, no studies of tDCS in youth with mood disorders have been published, although ongoing trials exist.[37] Study design, population characteristics, findings, and adverse effects (AEs) of published pediatric tDCS studies are described in **Table 1**. Details of stimulation parameters for each study is summarized in **Table 2**.

Schizophrenia

Mattai and colleagues[35] examined the tolerability of tDCS in 13 inpatient participants with COS treated concurrently with clozapine. Participants (aged 10–17 years) were assigned to 1 of 2 electrode placements based on predominant symptoms: anodes over bilateral dorsolateral prefrontal cortices (DLPFCs) to improve cognition ($n = 8$), or cathodes over bilateral superior temporal gyri to improve hallucinations ($n = 5$). Participants were randomized to active versus sham sessions; those assigned to sham were offered an additional 10 sessions of active open-label treatment. Participants received 2-mA stimulation in 10 20-minute sessions over 2 weeks. Before and after tDCS, participants underwent physical evaluation, electroencephalography (EEG), electrocardiography, and MRI, in addition to neurocognitive testing and mental status evaluation.

Active tDCS was associated with tingling (46.1%), itching (53.8%), transient skin erythema (30.7%), and fatigue (30.7%). Although 1 participant withdrew for reasons unrelated to tDCS, none terminated participation because of AEs. No clinical deterioration occurred on any physical or cognitive measure. Moreover, participants receiving sham stimulation reported AEs at comparable rates, although the investigators noted that the study lacked power to detect AE differences between conditions. Nonetheless, this study provided early evidence for tolerability in a clinical youth population. Although the investigators proposed further study of tDCS for mitigation of cognitive symptoms in COS, additional research has not been published to date.

Autism

In an open-label trial, Schneider and Hopp[36] examined the effect of tDCS on language acquisition in minimally verbal children with ASD. Ten participants aged 6 to 21 years received 2-mA stimulation in a single 30-minute session. The anode was placed over the left DLPFC and the cathode over the right supraorbital (SO) area, targeting Broca's area to enhance language acquisition. Vocabulary and syntax acquisition were measured with the Bilingual Aphasia Test before and after tDCS. The investigators found significant improvement and large effect sizes in vocabulary and syntax scores ($P = .007, d = 0.96$ and $P<.0005, d = 2.78$, respectively). tDCS was well-tolerated, and all participants completed the protocol without reported AEs.

Amatachaya and colleagues[33] applied tDCS to 20 young (aged 5-8 years) boys with ASD recruited from special education centers. In their first study, the investigators used a double-blind, randomized, sham-controlled, crossover approach with a

Table 1
Transcranial direct current stimulation studies in psychiatric conditions in children and adolescents

Study	Design	n Receiving Active tDCS (n ≤ 21y)	Age Range (y)	Diagnosis	Main Findings	Adverse Events/Effects
Autism						
Schneider & Hopp,[36] 2011	Open-label	10	6–21	ASD, language disorder	Improved syntax acquisition after tDCS	None
Amatachaya et al,[33] 2014	Double-blind, randomized, sham-controlled crossover	20	5–8	ASD	Improved autism symptoms (social, behavioral, sensory/cognitive, overall ATEC scores; CARS) and functioning (CGAS) with active tDCS compared to sham	None
Andrade et al,[18] 2014	Open-label	14	5–12	ASD, learning disorder, expressive language disorder, ADHD	tDCS feasible, well-tolerated in children with language and neurodevelopmental disorders	Mood changes, irritability, tingling, itching, burning sensation, headache, localized redness, sleepiness, trouble concentrating, scalp pain
Amatachaya et al,[34] 2015	Double-blind, randomized, sham-controlled crossover	20	5–8	ASD	Improved autism symptoms (social, behavioral ATEC scores) and increased EEG peak alpha frequency with active tDCS compared to sham	Transient erythematous rash
Costanzo et al,[28] 2015	Open-label (case report)	1	14	ASD, catatonia, mild intellectual disability	Reduction in total catatonia symptoms; complete recovery of eating and drinking; improvement maintained at 1 mo	Not reported

Study	Design	N	Age	Diagnosis	Outcome	Adverse effects
D'Urso et al,[29] 2015	Open-label	12 (9 ≤ 21y)	18–26	ASD, intellectual disability	Reduced irritability/aggression, social withdrawal, hyperactivity/noncompliance, and total ABC scores after tDCS	Transient, localized skin irritation; 2 participants discontinued due to inability to tolerate protocol
ADHD						
Prehn-Kristensen et al,[21] 2014	Double-blind, randomized, sham-controlled crossover	12	10–14	ADHD	Active tDCS improved memory consolidation (comparable to 12 healthy control comparators); active tDCS enhanced slow oscillations compared to sham	No effect on mood or alertness
Munz et al,[22] 2015	Double-blind, randomized, sham-controlled crossover	14	10–14	ADHD	Enhanced slow oscillations and reduced reaction time (improved behavioral inhibition) with active tDCS compared to sham	None
Soltaninejad et al,[26] 2015	Single-blind, randomized, sham-controlled crossover	20	15–17	ADHD	No effect of tDCS on interference inhibition (Stroop); increased accuracy of No-Go responses with left DLPFC cathodal stimulation; increased accuracy of Go responses with left DLPFC anodal stimulation	Not reported
Bandeira et al,[19] 2016	Open-label	9	7–15	ADHD	Improvement in some measures of visual attention and inhibitory control	Headache, neck pain, tingling, itching, burning sensation, localized redness, sleepiness, shocking sensation

(continued on next page)

Table 1
(continued)

Study	Design	n Receiving Active tDCS (n ≤ 21y)	Age Range (y)	Diagnosis	Main Findings	Adverse Events/Effects
Breitling et al,[23] 2016	Single-blind, pseudo-randomized/counterbalanced crossover	42 (21 ADHD, 21 healthy controls)	13–17	ADHD, healthy controls	Lower commission error rates and reaction time variability on modified Flanker task in ADHD patients receiving right IFG anodal tDCS compared to sham, with ADHD participants who received right IFG anodal stimulation having performance comparable to controls; no difference between right IFG cathodal and sham stimulation in either group	Skin irritation/sensations; no difference between active tDCS and sham for concentration
Nejati et al,[27] 2017	Double-blind, randomized, sham-controlled crossover Experiment 1: active tDCS (left DLPFC anodal/right DLPFC cathodal) vs sham Experiment 2: Montage 1 (left DLPFC anodal/right OFC cathodal) vs Montage 2 (right OFC anodal/left DLPFC cathodal) vs sham	25 Experiment 1: n = 15 Experiment 2: n = 10	7–15	ADHD	Experiment 1: No improvement inhibitory control, task switching, cognitive flexibility, or working memory with tDCS; reaction time, response inhibition improved with tDCS compared to sham Experiment 2: Improved response inhibition (No-Go accuracy) and executive function with Montage 2 compared to sham; both Montage 1 and 2 improved errors on WCST compared to sham; Montage 1 improved working memory compared	Itching, tingling

Study	Study design	N	Age	Diagnosis	Results	Adverse events
Soff et al,[24] 2017	Double-blind, randomized, sham-controlled crossover	15	12–16	ADHD	Improvement in inattention symptom scales with tDCS compared to sham; reduced hyperactivity and inattention on QbTest with tDCS compared to sham	Tingling, itching, headache; no difference in AEs between active tDCS and sham
Sotnikova et al,[25] 2017	Double-blind, randomized, sham-controlled crossover	16	12–16	ADHD	Active tDCS reduced reaction time and variability, but increased omission errors and reduced accuracy, compared to sham; active tDCS increased BOLD signal in left DLPFC, SMA, precuneus, and premotor cortex during working memory task compared to sham; active tDCS increased resting state functional connectivity of the left DLPFC and working memory networks compared to sham	Tingling, itching, headache, anxiety; no difference between active tDCS and sham
Learning Disorders						
Costanzo et al,[31] 2016	Double-blind, sham-controlled crossover (4 conditions)	19	10–17	Dyslexia	Reduced reading errors with left parietotemporal anodal/right parietotemporal cathodal active tDCS; increased errors with right parietotemporal anodal/left parietotemporal cathodal active tDCS	Tingling, itching, mild burning sensation, sleepiness

(continued on next page)

Table 1
(continued)

Study	Design	n Receiving Active tDCS (n ≤ 21y)	Age Range (y)	Diagnosis	Main Findings	Adverse Events/Effects
Costanzo et al,[30] 2016	Double-blind, randomized, sham-controlled	18 (active tDCS: 9)	10–17	Dyslexia	Reduced reading errors and increased reading speed with active tDCS compared to sham; improvements persistent at 1 mo	Tingling, itching, burning sensation, localized redness
Costanzo et al,[32] 2018	Double-blind, randomized, sham-controlled	26 (active tDCS: 13)	10–17	Dyslexia	Non-word reading efficiency and low-frequency word reading efficiency improved at 1- and 6-mo follow-up with active tDCS compared to sham	Transient tingling, itching; burning sensation, and local redness
Eating Disorders						
Khedr et al,[20] 2014	Open-label	7 (4 ≤ 21y)	16–39	AN	Improvement in AN and depression symptom scales after tDCS and 1-mo post-stimulation	Transient, localized itching
Psychotic Disorders						
Mattai et al,[35] 2011	Double-blind, randomized to active vs sham; assigned electrode placement based on symptoms; subsequent open-label phase for those initially receiving sham	13	10–17	COS	Well-tolerated in COS population; no changes in mood, mental status, vital signs, MRI, EEG, ECG	Transient redness, tingling, itching, fatigue; no statistically significant difference in AEs observed between active and sham tDCS

Abbreviations: ABC, Aberrant Behavior Checklist; ADHD, attention-deficit hyperactivity disorder; AE, adverse effect/event; AN, anorexia nervosa; ASD, autism spectrum disorder; ATEC, Autism Treatment Evaluation Checklist; BOLD, blood oxygen level-dependent; CARS, Childhood Autism Rating Scale; CGAS, Children's Global Assessment Scale; COS, childhood-onset schizophrenia; DLPFC, dorsolateral prefrontal cortex; ECG, electrocardiography; EEG, electroencephalography; fMRI, functional magnetic resonance imaging; IFG, inferior frontal gyrus; MRI, magnetic resonance imaging; OFC, orbitofrontal cortex; QBTest, Quantified behavior Test

Table 2
Stimulation parameters of child and adolescent psychiatric tDCS studies

Study	Electrode Placement[a]	Electrode Surface Area (cm²)	Current Intensity (mA)	Session Duration (min)	Current Density (mA/cm²)	Charge Density, per Session (C/m²)	Number of Sessions and Frequency	Concurrent Task
Autism								
Schneider & Hopp,[36] 2011	A: left DLPFC (F3) C: right SO	25	2.0	30	0.08	1440	1 session	Syntax training
Amatachaya et al,[33] 2014	A: left DLPFC (F3) C: right shoulder	35	1.0	20	0.029	348	5 sessions (1 session/day, 5 consecutive days/condition, crossover with 4-wk washout between conditions)	None
Andrade et al,[18] 2014	A: Broca's Area (F5) C: right SO (Fp2)	35	2.0	30	0.057	1026	10 sessions (1 session/day, 5 consecutive days/week, 2 wk)	Speech/social activities
Amatachaya et al,[34] 2015	A: left DLPFC (F3) C: right shoulder	35	1.0	20	0.029	348	1 session/condition (crossover with 1-wk washout between conditions)	None
Costanzo et al,[28] 2015	A: left DLPFC (F3) C: right DLPFC (F4)	25	1.0	20	0.04	480	28 sessions (1 session/day, 28 consecutive weekdays)	None
D'Urso et al,[29] 2015	A: right lateral arm C: left DLPFC (F3)	A: 40 C: 25	1.5	20	A: 0.038 C: 0.06	A: 456 C: 720	10 sessions (1 session/day, 5 d/wk, 2 wk)	Routine activities in occupational rehabilitation program

(continued on next page)

Table 2
(continued)

Study	Electrode Placement[a]	Electrode Surface Area (cm^2)	Current Intensity (mA)	Session Duration (min)	Current Density (mA/cm^2)	Charge Density, per Session (C/m^2)	Number of Sessions and Frequency	Concurrent Task
ADHD								
Prehn-Kristensen et al,[21] 2014	A: bilateral frontolateral (F3, F4) C: bilateral mastoid (M1, M2)	0.503	0.25 (peak current, oscillating at 0.75 Hz)	5 min × 5 blocks; 1 min between blocks	0.497 (peak)	Not reported (oscillating current)	1 session/condition (crossover with ≥1-wk washout between conditions)	Sleep
Munz et al,[22] 2015	A: bilateral frontolateral (F3, F4) C: bilateral mastoid (M1, M2)	0.503	0.25 (peak current, oscillating at 0.75 Hz)	5 min × 5 blocks; 1 min between blocks	0.497 (peak)	Not reported (oscillating current)	1 session/condition (crossover with ≥1-wk washout between conditions)	Sleep
Soltaninejad et al,[26] 2015	Condition 1: A: left DLPFC (F3) C: right SO (Fp2) Condition 2: A: right SO (Fp2) C: left DLPFC (F3) Condition 3: Sham stimulation	35	1.5	15	0.043	387	1 session/condition (crossover with 72-h washout between conditions)	Go/No-Go and Stroop tasks
Bandeira et al,[19] 2016	A: left DLPFC (F3) C: right SO (Fp2)	35	2.0	30	0.057	1026	5 sessions (1 session/day, 5 consecutive days)	Visual matching game
Breitling et al,[23] 2016	Condition 1: A: right IFG (F8) C: left mastoid Condition 2: A: left mastoid C: right IFG (F8) Condition 3: Sham stimulation	35	1.0	20	0.029	348	1 session/condition (crossover with ≥1-wk washout between conditions)	Modified Flanker task

	Montage					Sessions	Outcome
Nejati et al,[27] 2017	Experiment 1: A: left DLPFC (F3) C: right DLPFC (F4) Experiment 2: Montage 1: A: left DLPFC (F3) C: right OFC (Fp2) Montage 2: A: right OFC (Fp2) C: left DLPFC (F3)	25	1.0	15	0.04	360	1 session/condition (crossover with 72-h washout between conditions)	None
Soff et al,[24] 2017	A: left DLPFC (F3) C: vertex (Cz)	A: 3.14 C: 12.5	1.0	20	A: 0.318 C: 0.08	A: 3816 C: 960	5 sessions (1 session/day, 5 consecutive days/condition, 2-wk washout between conditions)	Quantified Behavior Test
Sotnikova et al,[25] 2017	A: left DLPFC (F3) C: vertex (Cz)	A: 13 C: 35	1.0	20	A: 0.077 C: 0.029	A: 924 C: 348	1 session/condition (crossover with 2-wk washout between conditions)	Quantified Behavior Test
Learning Disorders							
Costanzo et al,[31] 2016	Montage 1: A: left parietotemporal (P7-TP7 midpoint) C: right parietotemporal (P8-TP8 midpoint) Montage 2: A: right parietotemporal C: left parietotemporal	25	1.0	20	0.04	480	1 session/condition (crossover with ≥24-h washout between each condition)	None

(continued on next page)

Table 2
(continued)

Study	Electrode Placement[a]	Electrode Surface Area (cm²)	Current Intensity (mA)	Session Duration (min)	Current Density (mA/cm²)	Charge Density, per Session (C/m²)	Number of Sessions and Frequency	Concurrent Task
Costanzo et al,[30] 2016	A: left parietotemporal (P7-TP7 midpoint) C: right parietotemporal (P8-TP8 midpoint)	25	1.0	20	0.04	480	18 sessions (3 sessions/ week, 6 wk)	Tachistoscopic presentation of verbal stimuli, phonic training
Costanzo et al,[32] 2018	A: left parietotemporal (P7-TP7 midpoint) C: right parietotemporal (P8-TP8 midpoint)	25	1.0	20	0.04	480	18 sessions (3 sessions/ week, 6 wk)	Tachistoscopic presentation of verbal stimuli, phonic training
Eating Disorders								
Khedr et al,[20] 2014	A: left DLPFC C: right arm	A: 24 C: 100	2.0	25	A: 0.083 C: 0.02	A: 1245 C: 300	10 sessions (1 session/ day, 5 d/wk, 2 wk)	None
Psychotic Disorders								
Mattai et al,[35] 2011	Montage 1 (n = 8): A: bilateral DLPFC (Fp1, Fp2) C: non-dominant forearm Montage 2 (n = 5): A: non-dominant forearm C: bilateral STG (T3, T4)	25	2.0	20	0.08	960	10 sessions (1 session/ day, 5 d/wk, 2 wk)	None

Abbreviations: A, anode; C, cathode; DLPFC, dorsolateral prefrontal cortex; fMRI, functional magnetic resonance imaging; IFG, inferior frontal gyrus; OFC, orbitofrontal cortex; SMA, supplementary motor area; SO, supraorbital; STG, superior temporal gyrus.
[a] Electrode placements as described in the original articles. Placements are also denoted by the International 10-20 system for electroencephalographic scalp

4-week washout between phases. Five daily, 20-minute sessions of 1-mA tDCS were delivered (anode: left DLPFC; cathode: right shoulder). Improvements on the Childhood Autism Rating Scale ($P<.001$), the Autism Treatment Evaluation Checklist (ATEC, $P<.001$), and the Children's Global Assessment Scale ($P = .042$) were observed following active tDCS but not sham. No AEs were reported by participants or observed by investigators.

In the same sample, the investigators examined the effect of a single tDCS session (previous parameters; sham-controlled crossover design) on EEG-measured peak alpha frequency (PAF) and its relationship to ASD symptoms.[34] In addition to increased frontal PAF and improvements on ATEC social and health and behavioral problems domains, there were significant correlations between immediate changes in PAF and changes from baseline to 7-day ATEC scores (social: $r = -0.47, P = .037$, health and behavioral problems: $r = -0.46, P = .039$), suggesting that frontal cortical activity may underlie changes in ASD symptoms observed with tDCS.

Andrade and colleagues[18] studied tolerability and feasibility in 14 children (aged 5–12 years) with various neurodevelopmental conditions, including ASD, language disorders, intellectual disability, and global dyspraxia. Participants underwent 10 open-label tDCS sessions over 2 weeks (2-mA, 30 minutes per session, anode: Broca's area, cathode: right SO) with social interaction and speech activities during stimulation. A structured questionnaire[38] was used to assess AEs. Mood changes (42.9%), irritability (35.7%), tingling (28.6%), and itching (28.6%) were the most commonly observed, and most AEs were deemed mild.

In an open-label pilot study, D'Urso and colleagues[29] evaluated impact of tDCS on hyperactivity and noncompliance in 12 youth (aged 18–26 years; 9 participants ≤21 years) with ASD, intellectual disability, and speech impairment. One participant had comorbid epilepsy, and another had Down syndrome. Stimulation (10 daily 20-minute sessions, 1.5-mA) was delivered with right arm anodal and left DLPFC cathodal placement, aiming to improve behavioral inhibition. Two participants withdrew following difficulty tolerating the procedures. Among study completers, decreases were observed on the Aberrant Behavior Checklist total score ($P = .002$) and hyperactivity and noncompliance ($P = .002$), social withdrawal ($P = .03$), and irritability ($P = .003$) subscales. The investigators posited that tDCS could augment rehabilitative therapies in autistic youth and could be used safely in patients with comorbid epilepsy.

Costanzo and colleagues[28] reported the case of a 14-year-old adolescent with ASD, intellectual disability, and benzodiazepine-resistant catatonia who responded to 28 daily sessions of tDCS (1-mA, anode: left DLPFC, cathode: right DLPFC, 20 minutes per session). The patient experienced a 30% overall reduction in catatonic symptoms, and improvements largely persisted at 1 month.

Eating Disorders

Khedr and colleagues[20] conducted the only currently published study of tDCS in adolescents with anorexia nervosa (AN). Of the sample of 7, 4 participants were 21 years of age or younger. The investigators administered 10 open-label sessions (2-mA, 25 minutes per session, anode: left DLPFC, cathode: right arm) over 2 weeks, reasoning that this montage might reduce right hemispheric hyperactivity previously observed in AN. There was a significant effect of time (measured at baseline, immediately posttreatment, and 1-month follow-up), with improvement noted on the Eating Attitudes Test ($P = .016$), Eating Disorders Inventory ($P = .018$), and Beck Depression Inventory ($P = .016$).

Learning Disorders and Dyslexia

Costanzo and colleagues[31] examined effects on reading accuracy, lexical decision-making, and verbal working memory in 19 youth with dyslexia aged 10 to 17 years. Bilateral parietotemporal cortices were targeted for their role in phonological processing. Participants underwent single 20-minute sessions of 4 experimental conditions (1-mA active left anodal and right cathodal, 1-mA active right anodal and left cathodal, sham stimulation, and baseline testing without tDCS) in counterbalanced order, with a 24-hour or greater washout between sessions. Reading accuracy improved after left anodal and right cathodal stimulation (compared with baseline, sham, and right anodal and left cathodal), whereas errors increased after the right anodal and left cathodal condition (compared with baseline, sham, and left anodal and right cathodal stimulation). No other reading-related changes were significant. AEs (somnolence and localized itching, tingling, and burning sensations) were mild and transient.

In their second experiment,[30] the investigators evaluated tDCS in a double-blind, sham-controlled trial involving a similar sample (18 youth aged 10–17 years). Participants received 3 20-minute stimulation sessions per week for 6 weeks, which was paired with concurrent cognitive training (presentation of verbal stimuli via tachistoscope and phonic training). Active tDCS consisted of 1-mA stimulation (anode: left parietotemporal, cathode: right parietotemporal). Both low-frequency word reading accuracy and nonword reading speed improved immediately after treatment and at 1-month follow-up with active stimulation but not with sham. AEs were mild (localized scalp irritation). Using the same tDCS parameters, the investigators replicated these findings in a double-blind, sham-controlled trial in 26 children and adolescents (aged 10–17 years).[32] Participants who received active tDCS demonstrated improved nonword and low-frequency word reading efficiency, whereas sham treatment evidenced no changes. Reading effects persisted at 6 months, and AEs (scalp irritation) were mild and transient.

Attention-Deficit Hyperactivity Disorder

A relatively large number of pediatric tDCS studies have focused on ADHD. Prehn-Kristensen and colleagues[21] conducted a sham-controlled crossover study, using 0.75 Hz transcranial oscillating direct current stimulation (toDCS) to induce slow oscillations in the frontolateral cortex in 12 children (aged 10–14 years) with ADHD during sleep. Active toDCS not only increased frontolateral slow oscillation power on polysomnography during stage 4 sleep ($P = .02$) but also improved sleep-dependent memory consolidation ($P = .004$) to the level of healthy controls. The investigators suggested that toDCS could enhance nighttime memory consolidation, augmenting the effects of daytime medications. The same group later examined effects of 0.75 Hz toDCS during sleep on daytime behavioral inhibition in 14 children (aged 10–14 years) with ADHD.[22] Reaction times were shorter (indicating improved inhibition) on a visuomotor Go/No-Go task following active toDCS compared to sham; alertness and motor memory were unchanged.

Soltaninejad and colleagues[26] examined effects of tDCS in 20 adolescents (aged 15–17 years) with ADHD in a single-blind, sham-controlled crossover study. Single sessions of 3 conditions were tested, separated by 72-hour washouts: active tDCS (1.5-mA, 15 minutes) with left DLPFC anodal and right SO cathodal placement, active tDCS with right SO anodal and left DLPFC cathodal placement, and sham stimulation. All participants completed Stroop and Go/No-Go response inhibition tasks concurrently with tDCS sessions. Right SO anodal and left DLPFC cathodal stimulation improved accuracy of No-Go responses, whereas left DLPFC anodal and right SO cathodal stimulation improved accuracy of Go responses. No effect on interference inhibition on the Stroop task was observed. The investigators postulated that transcallosal connections may underlie these observed improvements in inhibition. Bandeira and colleagues[19] found that 5 30-minute sessions of 2-mA tDCS (anode: left DLPFC, cathode: right SO) improved certain measures of visual attention and inhibitory control in an open-label study of 9 youth (aged 7–15 years) with ADHD. Together, these findings suggest potential applications of tDCS to improve executive function and behavioral inhibition in children and adolescents with ADHD.

Breitling and colleagues[23] conducted a large trial of 21 adolescents (aged 13–17 years) with ADHD and 21 healthy control adolescents. Participants received single sessions of tDCS (1-mA, 20 minutes) in 3 conditions (sham; right inferior frontal gyrus anodal and left mastoid cathodal; and left mastoid anodal and right inferior frontal gyrus cathodal), with each session 1 week apart, while performing a modified Flanker test. ADHD patients receiving sham had greater commission error rates and reaction time variability compared with healthy controls. ADHD patients receiving anodal stimulation to the right inferior frontal gyrus showed fewer errors and reduced reaction time variability, equivalent to controls' performance.

Nejati and colleagues[27] conducted 2 experiments in a sample of 25 youth (aged 7–15 years) with ADHD. The first experiment compared performance on inhibition and executive function measures (Go/No-Go, Stroop, N-back, and Wisconsin Card Sorting Task) before and after a single 15-minute tDCS session (1-mA, anode: left DLPFC, cathode: right DLPFC). Anodal stimulation of the left DLPFC did not improve inhibitory control, cognitive flexibility, task switching, or number of accurate responses; however, it did reduce response time and improved interference response inhibition. The second experiment compared three conditions: left DLPFC anodal and right orbitofrontal cortex (OFC) cathodal stimulation; right OFC anodal and left DLPFC cathodal stimulation; and sham stimulation. They found that right OFC anodal and left DLPFC cathodal stimulation significantly increased response inhibition compared with sham, whereas both active stimulation paradigms significantly reduced perseverative errors compared with sham. Additionally, left DLPFC anodal and right OFC cathodal stimulation improved working memory performance compared with right OFC anodal and left DLPFC cathodal stimulation and sham in this ADHD population.

Another group administered anodal 1-mA tDCS to the left DLPFC in adolescents (aged 12–16 years) with ADHD in a randomized, double-blind, sham-controlled crossover study involving 5 20-minute sessions over 1 week ($n = 15$),[24] and single 20-minute tDCS sessions in conjunction with task-based and resting-state functional MRI (fMRI; $n = 16$).[25] After a 2-week washout, participants underwent the alternate treatment condition. ADHD symptoms, cognitive performance, and motor behavior were measured. Active tDCS significantly improved inattention and hyperactivity at one week post-stimulation ($P < .05$). tDCS was well-tolerated despite high anodal charge density (3816 C/m^2). Task-based fMRI found that anodal tDCS increased blood oxygen level–dependent signals in the left DLPFC, left premotor and supplementary motor cortices, and right precuneus, suggesting that stimulation increased neural activity during a concurrent working memory task. Resting-state fMRI found increased global connectivity in the left DLPFC after tDCS.[25]

ADVERSE EFFECTS IN CHILDREN AND ADOLESCENTS

AEs in individual pediatric studies have generally been minor and transient. A systematic review of safety and tolerability in tDCS and other transcranial electrical stimulation identified 14 pediatric tDCS studies and 2 studies using transcranial alternating current stimulation, with a total of 191 youth aged 2 to 17 years.[1] All studies except 1 provided AE information. Reported AEs included tingling sensations (incidence 11.5%), itching (5.8%), skin erythema (4.7%), scalp discomfort (3.1%), mood changes (3.1%), fatigue (2.1%), headache (1.0%), burning sensations (1.0%), and sleepiness (1.0%). No studies reported severe AEs or delayed onset of AEs. No AEs necessitated medical intervention. Although the investigators concluded that the available pediatric literature indicated good safety and tolerability, they recommended that future studies track the occurrence of AEs in a systematic, quantitative, and active manner. Additionally, studies with longer follow-up periods will be necessary to establish long-term safety.[1]

FUTURE DIRECTIONS IN PEDIATRIC TRANSCRANIAL DIRECT CURRENT STIMULATION RESEARCH

tDCS research in children and adolescents is still in its infancy, and recommendations regarding routine clinical application would be premature. However, it is an active area of research, with 13 active and 4 recently completed trials enrolling children and adolescents listed in the ClinicalTrials.gov registry. Ongoing studies are investigating tDCS in a wide range of psychiatric conditions in youth, including depression, obsessive-compulsive disorder, tic disorders, eating disorders, neurodevelopmental disorders (ADHD, fetal alcohol spectrum, and ASD), early-onset psychosis, impulse-control disorders, suicidality, and comorbid medical and psychiatric conditions.[37]

In summary, tDCS research is a young but rapidly developing field, with substantial promise for research and clinical applications. Preliminary evidence in children and adolescents suggests short-term safety and tolerability, as well as encouraging effects on some clinical symptoms. However, large randomized controlled trials providing definitive efficacy data are lacking in youth. Additionally, the incomplete knowledge of how stimulation interacts with the developing brain and how tDCS affects learning and task enhancement in children and adolescents demands substantial caution. Much further research is necessary before tDCS can be considered an evidence-based therapeutic intervention for youth with psychiatric conditions.

REFERENCES

1. Krishnan C, Santos L, Peterson MD, et al. Safety of noninvasive brain stimulation in children and adolescents. Brain Stimul 2015;8(1):76–87.
2. Muszkat D, Polanczyk GV, Dias TG, et al. Transcranial direct current stimulation in child and adolescent psychiatry. J Child Adolesc Psychopharmacol 2016;26(7):590–7.
3. Palm U, Segmiller FM, Epple AN, et al. Transcranial direct current stimulation in children and adolescents: a comprehensive review. J Neural Transm 2016;123(10):1219–34.
4. Lee JC, Lewis CP, Daskalakis ZJ, et al. Transcranial direct current stimulation: considerations for research in adolescent depression. Front Psychiatry 2017;8:91.
5. Rivera-Urbina GN, Nitsche MA, Vicario CM, et al. Applications of transcranial direct current stimulation in children and pediatrics. Rev Neurosci 2017;28(2):173–84.
6. Silverstein FS, Jensen FE. Neonatal seizures. Ann Neurol 2007;62(2):112–20.
7. Duncan CE, Webster MJ, Rothmond DA, et al. Prefrontal GABA$_A$ receptor α-subunit expression in normal postnatal human development and schizophrenia. J Psychiatr Res 2010;44(10):673–81.

8. Rakhade SN, Jensen FE. Epileptogenesis in the immature brain: emerging mechanisms. Nat Rev Neurol 2009;5(7):380–91.

9. Ben-Ari Y, Khazipov R, Leinekugel X, et al. GABA$_A$, NMDA and AMPA receptors: a developmentally regulated 'ménage à trois. Trends Neurosci 1997;20(11): 523–9.

10. Leinekugel X, Khalilov I, McLean H, et al. GABA is the principal fast-acting excitatory transmitter in the neonatal brain. In: Delgado-Escueta AV, Wilson WA, Olsen RW, et al, editors. Jasper's basic mechanisms of the epilepsies, thirrd edition: advances in neurology, vol. 79. Philadelphia: Lippincott Williams & Wilkins; 1999. p. 189–201.

11. Koerte I, Heinen F, Fuchs T, et al. Anisotropy of callosal motor fibers in combination with transcranial magnetic stimulation in the course of motor development. Invest Radiol 2009;44(5):279–84.

12. Moliadze V, Schmanke T, Andreas S, et al. Stimulation intensities of transcranial direct current stimulation have to be adjusted in children and adolescents. Clin Neurophysiol 2015;126(7):1392–9.

13. Beauchamp MS, Beurlot MR, Fava E, et al. The developmental trajectory of brain-scalp distance from birth through childhood: implications for functional neuroimaging. PLoS One 2011;6(9):e24981.

14. Minhas P, Bikson M, Woods AJ, et al. Transcranial direct current stimulation in pediatric brain: a computational modeling study. Conf Proc IEEE Eng Med Biol Soc 2012;2012:859–62.

15. Kessler SK, Minhas P, Woods AJ, et al. Dosage considerations for transcranial direct current stimulation in children: a computational modeling study. PLoS One 2013;8(9):e76112.

16. Liebetanz D, Koch R, Mayenfels S, et al. Safety limits of cathodal transcranial direct current stimulation in rats. Clin Neurophysiol 2009;120(6):1161–7.

17. Bikson M, Grossman P, Thomas C, et al. Safety of transcranial direct current stimulation: evidence based update 2016. Brain Stimul 2016;9(5):641–61.

18. Andrade AC, Magnavita GM, Allegro JV, et al. Feasibility of transcranial direct current stimulation use in children aged 5 to 12 years. J Child Neurol 2014; 29(10):1360–5.

19. Bandeira ID, Guimarães RSQ, Jagersbacher JG, et al. Transcranial direct current stimulation in children and adolescents with attention-deficit/hyperactivity disorder (ADHD): a pilot study. J Child Neurol 2016;31(7):918–24.

20. Khedr EM, Elfetoh NA, Ali AM, et al. Anodal transcranial direct current stimulation over the dorsolateral prefrontal cortex improves anorexia nervosa: a pilot study. Restor Neurol Neurosci 2014;32(6):789–97.

21. Prehn-Kristensen A, Munz M, Göder R, et al. Transcranial oscillatory direct current stimulation during sleep improves declarative memory consolidation in children with attention-deficit/hyperactivity disorder to a level comparable to healthy controls. Brain Stimul 2014;7(6):793–9.

22. Munz MT, Prehn-Kristensen A, Thielking F, et al. Slow oscillating transcranial direct current stimulation during non-rapid eye movement sleep improves behavioral inhibition in attention-deficit/hyperactivity disorder. Front Cell Neurosci 2015; 9:307.

23. Breitling C, Zaehle T, Dannhauer M, et al. Improving interference control in ADHD patients with transcranial direct current stimulation (tDCS). Front Cell Neurosci 2016;10:72.

24. Soff C, Sotnikova A, Christiansen H, et al. Transcranial direct current stimulation improves clinical symptoms in adolescents with attention deficit hyperactivity disorder. J Neural Transm 2017;124(1):133–44.

25. Sotnikova A, Soff C, Tagliazucchi E, et al. Transcranial direct current stimulation modulates neuronal networks in attention deficit hyperactivity disorder. Brain Topogr 2017;30(5):656–72.

26. Soltaninejad Z, Nejati V, Ekhtiari H. Effect of anodal and cathodal transcranial direct current stimulation on DLPFC on modulation of inhibitory control in ADHD. J Atten Disord 2015. [Epub ahead of print].

27. Nejati V, Salehinejad MA, Nitsche MA, et al. Transcranial direct current stimulation improves executive dysfunctions in ADHD: implications for inhibitory control, interference control, working memory, and cognitive flexibility. J Atten Disord 2017. [Epub ahead of print].

28. Costanzo F, Menghini D, Casula L, et al. Transcranial direct current stimulation treatment in an adolescent with autism and drug-resistant catatonia. Brain Stimul 2015;8(6):1233–5.

29. D'Urso G, Bruzzese D, Ferrucci R, et al. Transcranial direct current stimulation for hyperactivity and noncompliance in autistic disorder. World J Biol Psychiatry 2015;16(5):361–6.

30. Costanzo F, Varuzza C, Rossi S, et al. Evidence for reading improvement following tDCS treatment in children and adolescents with dyslexia. Restor Neurol Neurosci 2016;34(2):215–26.

31. Costanzo F, Varuzza C, Rossi S, et al. Reading changes in children and adolescents with dyslexia after transcranial direct current stimulation. Neuroreport 2016; 27(5):295–300.

32. Costanzo F, Rossi S, Varuzza C, et al. Long-lasting improvement following tDCS treatment combined with a training for reading in children and adolescents with dyslexia. Neuropsychologia 2018. [Epub ahead of print].

33. Amatachaya A, Auvichayapat N, Patjanasoontorn N, et al. Effect of anodal transcranial direct current stimulation on autism: a randomized double-blind crossover trial. Behav Neurol 2014;2014:173073.

34. Amatachaya A, Jensen MP, Patjanasoontorn N, et al. The short-term effects of transcranial direct current stimulation on electroencephalography in children with autism: a randomized crossover controlled trial. Behav Neurol 2015;2015: 928631.

35. Mattai A, Miller R, Weisinger B, et al. Tolerability of transcranial direct current stimulation in childhood-onset schizophrenia. Brain Stimul 2011;4(4):275–80.

36. Schneider HD, Hopp JP. The use of the Bilingual Aphasia Test for assessment and transcranial direct current stimulation to modulate language acquisition in minimally verbal children with autism. Clin Linguist Phon 2011;25(6–7):640–54.

37. U.S. National Library of Medicine. ClinicalTrials.gov. 2018. Available at: https:// clinicaltrials.gov. Accessed May 17, 2018.

38. Brunoni AR, Amadera J, Berbel B, et al. A systematic review on reporting and assessment of adverse effects associated with transcranial direct current stimulation. Int J Neuropsychopharmacol 2011;14(8):1133–45.

Anti-N-Methyl D-Aspartate Receptor Encephalitis and Electroconvulsive Therapy
Literature Review and Future Directions

Yasas Chandra Tanguturi, MBBS, MPH, Allyson Witters Cundiff, MD,
Catherine Fuchs, MD*

KEYWORDS

- Electroconvulsive therapy • ECT • Anti-NMDA encephalitis
- Autoimmune encephalitis • Catatonia

KEY POINTS

- Catatonia is a syndrome, with one potential cause being an autoimmune encephalitis such as anti-N-methyl D-aspartate receptor encephalitis.
- Benzodiazepines (BZDs) are first-line treatment for symptoms of the syndrome of catatonia.
- Electroconvulsive therapy (ECT) should be considered if patients have autonomic instability or if they are not responding well to BZDs in combination with immunotherapy. The use of BZDs + ECT may be synergistic in efficacy.
- ECT is considered a safe intervention with appropriate assessment and management, although the exact mechanism of action of ECT is unclear.
- Treatment should be a multidisciplinary collaborative effort to include assessment and treatment of the autoimmune process.

INTRODUCTION

Anti-N-methyl D-aspartate receptor (NMDAR) encephalitis is an autoimmune encephalitis caused by the binding of antibodies to extracellular epitopes of cell-surface proteins of the receptor causing reversible neuronal dysfunction. It is the most commonly identified autoimmune encephalitis.[1] Dalmau first described the implicated antibodies to the GluN1 (NR1) subunit of the NMDAR in 2007.[2] Confirmatory diagnosis requires detection of these in the cerebrospinal fluid (CSF); serum testing can be done but

Disclosure Statement: The authors have no conflicts of interest to disclose.
Village at Vanderbilt, Suite 2200, 1500 21st Avenue South, Nashville, TN 37212, USA
* Corresponding author.
E-mail address: catherine.fuchs@vanderbilt.edu

Child Adolesc Psychiatric Clin N Am 28 (2019) 79–89
https://doi.org/10.1016/j.chc.2018.07.005
1056-4993/19/© 2018 Elsevier Inc. All rights reserved.

childpsych.theclinics.com

has a 14% false-negative rate.[1] NMDA receptors are important for synaptic transmission and plasticity, with the NR1 subunits binding glycine and the NR2 subunits binding glutamate. NMDA-receptor antagonists such as ketamine and phencyclidine can cause symptoms that mimic NMDA encephalitis. The effect on the NMDA receptors is reversed when antibodies are removed in vitro.[3]

Similar to other causes of autoimmune encephalitis, identified triggers for anti-NMDAR encephalitis include tumors and viral infections.[1] The condition primarily affects children and young adults with median age of 21 years (range 2 months–85 years). It is more common in women when younger (a ratio of 4:1) but equalizes after the age of 45 years. Up to 58% of women have an ovarian teratoma,[1] with the tumor being more commonly detected in women older than 18 years.[4] Clinical features of anti-NMDAR encephalitis have also been well described in the literature.[3,4] Children typically present with neurologic symptoms such as seizures and movement abnormalities in addition to insomnia, behavioral changes, and decreased verbalization; adults typically present with psychiatric and behavioral symptoms.[1,5] Two clinical stages have been detailed,[6,7] with the first stage characterized by a prodromal nonspecific virallike illness approximately 2 weeks before admission to a hospital. The course then proceeds to psychiatric symptoms including anxiety, agitation, bizarre behavior, delusional or paranoid thoughts, and visual or auditory hallucinations. Most of the patients also have seizures and alterations in level of consciousness.

The vast majority of patients (84%) have motor symptoms consistent with a catatonic syndrome during the course of the illness.[3] Various symptoms have been identified in the literature, including akinesis alternating with agitation, decreased or paradoxic responses to stimuli such as pain, changes in speech patterns and frequency including echolalia or mutism, staring, dyskinesias, autonomic instability, and central hypoventilation. A subset of patients has also been documented to have cardiac dysrhythmias. The most frequent catatonic symptoms include orofacial dyskinesias.[3,4] Although it is hypothesized that in some patients the catatonia might be related to antipsychotic use, the consistency of catatonic symptoms in presentation seems to indicate they are related to the disease process itself.[8] Anti-NMDAR encephalitis also seems to increase the risk of neuroleptic malignant syndrome with use of antipsychotics.[1]

TREATMENT OF ANTI-N-METHYL D-ASPARTATE RECEPTOR ENCEPHALITIS

Since the disorder is thought to be an immune response within the central nervous system, discussion of treatment in the literature has often focused on various forms of immunotherapy. In those patients who have a detectable tumor, surgical removal has been shown to be effective in treatment,[9] likely due to loss of the trigger for antibody production. Immunotherapy has been hypothesized to manage the effect of the antibody on the receptors as well as decreasing antibody production.[10] Response to first-line immunotherapy such as corticosteroids, plasma exchange, and intravenous immunoglobulins (IVIG) is often slow[9]; additional response may be obtained with the addition of second-line agents such as rituximab, cyclophosphamide, or both. One complicating factor is that the antibodies targeted are behind the blood-brain barrier, which may affect the effectiveness of plasma exchange or IVIG.[1] Symptoms may also relapse; it has been hypothesized that commonly used immunotherapies do not result in rapid and sustained control of the immune process.[3] Recovery can take up to 2 years. In one study of 577 patients receiving immunotherapy, only 53% improved clinically in 4 weeks with 81% recovering significantly at 24 months.[5] Median time from presentation to initial symptom improvement is estimated to be about 6 weeks (range 2–28 weeks),[4] with many patients requiring management in medical intensive care units.

Limited information exists within the literature on treatments traditionally used for catatonia symptoms such as autonomic instability and hypoventilation syndromes. There are no studies that have demonstrated the use of benzodiazepines (BZDs) or electroconvulsive therapy (ECT) in anti-NMDAR encephalitis presenting with catatonia. This may be because of a lack of understanding catatonia as a syndrome that may be associated with NMDAR encephalitis.

THE SYNDROME OF CATATONIA

Decisions regarding the treatment of anti-NMDAR encephalitis presenting with catatonic features necessitate an understanding of catatonia cause and pathophysiology. Catatonia was initially described in 1874 by Karl Kahlbaum as a subtype of dementia praecox. This led to classification of catatonia as a subtype of schizophrenia as defined in the Diagnostic and Statistical Manual of Mental Disorders (DSM)-III-R.[11] With improved understanding catatonia has been reconceptualized as a syndrome of neuropsychiatric symptoms with multiple potential causes, including metabolic, neurologic, toxic, and psychiatric conditions,[12] as well as autoimmune causes.[13] The DSM-IV identified 3 subtypes of catatonia: (1) schizophrenia, (2) affective disorders, and (3) medical conditions.[14] The DSM-V created a separate category of catatonia: (1) associated with another medical condition, (2) due to another mental disorder, and (3) unspecified.[15] Recent research posits a molecular hypothesis for a shared pathway to explain similarities of catatonic symptoms in a wide variety of illnesses (psychiatric disorders, neurologic diseases, general medical conditions, and genetic/immune disorders or exposure to toxins).[16] One hypothesis is that catatonia is the end result of nucleolar dysfunction due to abnormalities in the brain-specific C/D box noncoding, small nucleolar ribonucleic acid, specifically the SNORD115 genes. It is postulated that these genes may affect combinations of downstream functions, thus explaining the wide range of clinical subtypes of catatonia.[16] Changes in the function of dopamine and abnormalities in the gamma-aminobutyric acid/glutamate systems[12] and increased NMDA receptor activity[13] have also been implicated. A broader understanding of catatonia is necessary to consider unique treatment characteristics while expanding on knowledge of general concepts of treatment in the literature.

ELECTROCONVULSIVE THERAPY FOR CATATONIA

ECT has been an accepted treatment of catatonia since the 1930s.[17] Morrison references 14 cases of patients with neurologic conditions who presented with catatonic symptoms leading to an inaccurate diagnosis of catatonic schizophrenia. A subset had a pattern of rapid symptom onset over days to 2 weeks. These were associated with encephalitis, hepatic failure or other toxicity, or vascular events. Others had symptoms lasting from weeks to years associated with other medical disorders such as subdural hematomas, hyperthyroidism, temporal lobe tumors, and arteriovenous malformations. Favorable responses were documented for ECT when used in life-threatening catatonia.[17] Although limited in understanding of the syndromic nature of catatonia or the interface with medical causes, the paper highlights a long-standing recognition of medical disorders presenting with catatonic symptoms and the utility of ECT. Multiple studies over the years have documented the effectiveness and safety of ECT for catatonia.[18–20]

In the literature on catatonia, the treatments with the most evidence include ECT and lorazepam (oral, intravenous, or intramuscular). A recent review of 31 studies[12] discussing the treatment of catatonia reveals a wide variation in lorazepam dose, ECT method (unilateral or bilateral), or combined treatment. Response to ECT ranged from 59% to 100%. Studies in which BZDs were administered at 2 to 2.5 mg per dose with dosing several times per day resulted in greater response and remission rates (doses of up to 36 mg per day for an adolescent have been documented in the literature[10]). In the review, chronic catatonia had a poorer response to lorazepam. ECT was recommended after 4 to 5 days of BZDs if there was an inadequate response. To the authors' knowledge there has not been a protocol developed in the literature that addresses the inclusion of ECT for treatment of catatonic syndromes resulting from autoimmune encephalitis.

REVIEW OF LITERATURE

The authors performed a search of the literature for articles looking at the use of ECT specifically in anti-NMDA receptor antibody–mediated encephalitis. They used the PubMed database and excluded any articles not in English. They also used cross-referencing to further identify articles of relevance. **Table 1** summarizes the treatment approaches and antibody confirmation status for the case reports reviewed later.

Coffey and Cooper[8] published a review of the literature in 2016. They identified 6 case reports[10,21–25] that document the use of ECT in anti-NMDAR encephalitis. Four of these patients were younger than 18 years. ECT was used specifically to treat catatonic symptoms in all of these cases. The investigators questioned whether the catatonic symptoms were due to the use of neuroleptic agents or a direct manifestation of the disease process itself. With the use of ECT, direct benefits were noted for improvement in hemodynamics, motor abnormalities, cognition, and behavior. The reports were significant for the concomitant use of other treatments—immunotherapy, other pharmacotherapy, and surgery, along with ECT. The number of ECT sessions administered ranged from 2 to 13. There was a great deal of variation in the timing of ECT administration (before diagnostic confirmation vs after). The authors reviewed each of these case reports with a specific focus on catatonia symptoms and details related to ECT parameters.

Braakman and colleagues[21] described the use of ECT in a 47-year-old man who developed extrapyramidal symptoms, catalepsy, mutism, and respiratory failure in addition to psychiatric symptoms. Lorazepam and steroids did not improve symptoms. ECT was then initiated. Seven bilateral ECT treatments were delivered with good improvement in consciousness, catatonia, and other extrapyramidal symptoms. They questioned the temporality of symptoms and improvement and considered whether the condition could have been self-limited. Only laterality of ECT was described.

Matsumoto and colleagues[22] treated an 18-year-old man who presented with symptoms of confusion, catalepsy, stereotypy, convulsions, and tongue movements in addition to behavioral abnormalities and personality changes. He was initially treated with antipsychotics, lorazepam, and sodium valproate with limited response. He did however improve with 13 sessions of ECT along with antipsychotics. Specific ECT characteristics are not described, and it is unclear which symptoms were most responsive to ECT.

Mann and colleagues[23] described the case of a 14-year-old girl who presented with acute auditory hallucinations and paranoia. She developed a generalized tonic-clonic seizure, waxing and waning mental status, word-finding difficulties, mutism, and other

Table 1
Treatments used simultaneously with ECT for anti-NMDAR encephalitis

	Braakman et al,[21] 2010	Matsumoto et al,[22] 2012	Mann et al,[23] 2012	Wilson et al,[10] 2013	Jones et al,[24] 2015	Sunwoo et al,[25] 2016	Lee et al,[26] 2006	Slooter et al,[27] 2005
Age/Gender	47/M	18/M	14/F	14/F	17/M	27/F	11/F	13/F
Antibody confirmation	+	+	+	+	+	+	–	–
Lorazepam	10 mg/d for 3 d (before ECT)	–	2 mg IV every 6 h (before ECT)	3 mg IV every 2 h (before & with ECT)	2 mg IV every 2 h for 2 doses and then as needed (before ECT)	–	0.5–2 mg as needed	7 mg/d
Steroids	+	+	+	+	–	–	–	–
IVIG	–	–	+	+	+	+	–	–
Rituximab	–	–	+	+	–	+	–	–
Plasmapheresis	–	–	+	–	–	–	–	–
AEDs	+	+	+	+	+	+	–	+
ECT	7 sessions bilateral	13 sessions	7 sessions	14 sessions	2 sessions bitemporal	12 sessions bitemporal	8 sessions bilateral	13 sessions bilateral
Tumor	–	–	–	+	–	+	+	–
Antipsychotics	–	+	+	+	+	+	+	–
Other tx	–	–	–	–	Memantine	Cisatracurium (self-injury)	Bromocriptine	Bromocriptine

Abbreviation: AED, automated external defibrillator.

catatonic symptoms. She was initially treated with prednisone, then risperidone, which worsened catatonic symptoms. Lorazepam improved symptoms, but because of autonomic instability, a course of 7 ECT treatments was initiated. ECT (performed almost 3 months after initial symptom onset) led to improvement in mental status, and she was able to perform self-care with assistance. She received further treatment with valproic acid, trazodone, plasma exchange, rituximab, and cyclophosphamide. Symptoms improved in 8 months. No description of ECT characteristics was provided.

Wilson and colleagues[10] published a case report of a 14-year-old girl presenting with catatonic symptoms of immobility, stupor, mutism, staring, grimacing, posturing and rigidity, autonomic instability (tachycardia, hypertension), and respiratory depression necessitating advanced life support. Bush Francis score was 21. High-dose steroids and 2 courses of immunoglobulin did not alter symptoms. Although there was some improvement in muscle rigidity on a high-dose lorazepam regimen, this was not sustained. She received 14 treatments of ECT. Notably, ECT decreased rigidity, which enabled the effective completion of an abdominal computed tomography (CT) and discovery of an ovarian teratoma. Symptoms continued to improve with tumor removal, ongoing ECT, rituximab, steroids, and lorazepam. Initially, ECT was administered daily with a gradual increase in interval; no other ECT characteristics were described.

Jones and colleagues[24] used ECT for a 17-year-old man who presented with new onset confusion, catatonia, and seizures. Symptoms included concerns for delirium with disorganized behavior and thought process, in addition to signs of catatonia (autonomic instability, decreased level of responsiveness, dystonia, posturing, purposeless movement, cataplexy, waxy flexibility, stereotypy, pressured speech, echolalia, and orofacial dyskinesia). The patient was treated with lorazepam (unclear for how long and maximal dosing) with reported minimal response. He also failed multiple antipsychotics including risperidone, haloperidol, olanzapine and quetiapine, as well as antiepileptics, and continued to have seizurelike episodes. ECT was initiated to treat catatonia due to failure of lorazepam and the patient received 2 treatments. Described ECT characteristics include electrode placement (bitemporal), seizure duration (47–91 seconds), and dose (pulse width of 1 ms, current of 0.8 mA, frequency 40 Hz, and duration of 2 seconds; frequency and duration were increased in second treatment to 60 Hz and 3 seconds, respectively). Good improvement was reported in autonomic instability, stereotyped behaviors, and agitation. Of note, ECT was stopped after 2 treatments because confirmation of anti-NMDA antibodies was obtained from CSF testing. The patient was then switched over to immunotherapy with gradual improvement. A commentary published in the same journal issue by Kahn noted similarities with other cases reported in the literature and substantial improvement with ECT. The investigator hypothesized that the addition of ECT could improve and hasten outcomes when compared with immunotherapy and/or tumor removal.

Sunwoo and colleagues[25] published a case report of a 27-year-old woman with protracted dyskinesia that was nonresponsive to immunotherapy. Initial presenting symptoms included headache, insomnia, confusion, audiovisual hallucinations, disorganized speech, and decrease in consciousness. In spite of early surgical removal of an ovarian teratoma, dystonic symptoms worsened. The level of dyskinesia was noteworthy and reportedly did not respond to benzodiazepines and 8 doses of rituximab, leading to neuromuscular blockade with cisatracurium. After failure of all other treatment approaches for a period of 5 months, ECT was initiated with dramatic improvement within 2 weeks. The patient received 12 treatments of biweekly ECT with improvements in dyskinesia and consciousness. Characteristics of ECT described include laterality (bitemporal), stimulus dose (192–432 mC), current (800 mA), and seizure duration (33–63 seconds). Of note, patient did not receive any additional neuromuscular blockade due to being on continuous cisatracurium.

The authors also reviewed 2 older case reports of patients not formally diagnosed with anti-NMDAR encephalitis but in whom there was a characteristic clinical presentation and documented use of ECT.

Lee and colleagues[26] published in 2006 a case report of an 11-year-old woman described as paraneoplastic limbic encephalitis with malignant catatonia. Presentation included speech difficulties, confusion, agitation, insomnia, and psychosis. Initial diagnosis of probable schizophrenia was treated with antipsychotics. She developed muscular rigidity, autonomic instability, catalepsy, purposeless movements, and mutism. Use of benzodiazepines was not mentioned. Eight sessions of ECT yielded rapid response within 2 weeks. Improvements were documented in catalepsy, rigidity, and cognitive ability (able to do mathematical problems and 7-digit number sequences). An ovarian teratoma was discovered on an abdominal CT scan (obtained for pain and obstipation) after the eighth ECT treatment leading to surgical removal. ECT characteristics were described for charge (105 increased to 30%), pulse width (0.25 ms), frequency (20 Hz to 50 Hz), stimulus duration (5.6–6.72 seconds) and seizure duration of at least 25 seconds.

Slooter and colleagues[27] published a case report of a 13-year-old woman in 2005 (before development of testing for anti-NMDA antibodies). The investigators used the terminology "malignant catatonia" for symptoms with a presumed cause of encephalitis of unknown origin. Symptoms at the onset of illness included headaches, myoclonic jerks, dysphasia, lowered level of consciousness evolving into akinetic mutism, staring, rigidity, agitation, and dystonia. Symptoms responded to 13 ECT sessions over a period of 1 month. Described ECT characteristics include electrode placement (bilateral), seizure duration (at least 20 seconds), pulse width (1 ms), pulse duration (3.2 seconds), current (0.75–0.92 mA), and frequency (30–70 Hz).

Treatment approaches vary widely within these published case reports. **Table 1** lists the various treatments documented. Medications used include benzodiazepines, antipsychotics, antiepileptics, memantine, carbidopa/levodopa, bromocriptine, and other medications in addition to ECT and/or immunotherapy. Of note, most patients received ECT only after other initial treatments had failed. Regardless of the presence or absence of a tumor, ECT was equally efficacious. In one case, ECT decreased rigidity, which led to the discovery of a tumor.[10] Most of these reports lacked clear descriptions of the procedural aspects of ECT. One report mentioned the difficulties of achieving a seizure while the patient was on lorazepam.[24] No other operational challenges were described. No adverse events from the ECT were documented in any of these patients, indicating a high degree of safety despite multiple risk factors.

MECHANISM OF ACTION

There is a limited recognition of ECT as an effective and safe component of treatment of anti-NMDAR encephalitis. This could be explained by a historical stigma against ECT.[18] The exact mechanisms of action of ECT's therapeutic effect are also not well understood, which may contribute to reluctance to use. Some evidence in the literature comes from neuropsychiatric aspects of autoimmune diseases such as systemic lupus erythematosus.[28] Singh and Kar[29] have proposed 3 theories for therapeutic effect of ECT: neurophysiologic, neurobiochemical, and neuroplasticity.

The neurophysiologic theory postulates ECT changes in electrical patterns in the brain can lead to alterations in cerebral blood flow and glucose metabolism. Ictal phase changes in blood pressure may alter blood-brain barrier activity, which may transform the microenvironment, including levels of brain-derived neurotropic factor (BDNF).

The neurobiochemical theory hypothesizes effects on neurotransmitter synthesis, release, and ability to bind to receptors as well as reuptake. It has been hypothesized that ECT could be effective in NMDA encephalitis through a direct action on upregulation of the NMDA receptor system mediated by tissue plasminogen activator.[30–32] In animals, ECT may act at the level of gene expression and alter levels of neurotropic factors, both in terms of neuronal proliferation and neuroprotection. ECT may stimulate immune and neurotrophic systems, increasing BDNF, which could lead to neurogenesis. Modulation of BDNF could be one of the mechanisms of action of ECT, given its neurotropic properties implicated in both immune illness and depression. ECT influences both the peripheral immune system and microglial cells (which manufacture BDNF), leading to increased gliogenesis and neurogenesis.

Although this effect is poorly understood, Singh and colleagues[29] also hypothesize that ECT may modify the functional connectivity of brain structures or changes in neuroplasticity. ECT has been reported as a potent inducer of hippocampal neuroplasticity, with arborization of dendrites and hippocampal cell formation, which may be dose-dependent.[31] ECT has been demonstrated in animal models to reduce dendritic arborization and excitatory synapses in the amygdala. These hippocampal and amygdala mechanisms may promote recovery.

These proposed mechanisms are hypotheses based on mostly animal models and some human studies. There continues to be a limited understanding of the action due to small study sizes, inconsistent research methodology, and lack of control groups.[29]

DISCUSSION OF ELECTROCONVULSIVE THERAPY AS AN INDICATED TREATMENT FOR ANTI-N-METHYL D-ASPARTATE RECEPTOR ENCEPHALITIS

In medicine, the standard of care typically includes treatment of the underlying cause of disorder while managing the clinical symptoms. The authors identify that catatonic symptomatology should be categorized as a syndrome with multiple causes, which includes anti-NMDAR encephalitis. Multiple medical causes have been known to present with catatonia including other forms of autoimmune encephalitis.[23] Using a syndromic treatment approach helps with both understanding the pathophysiology and identifying a consistent paradigm.

As evidenced in our literature search, there is only limited information from case reports about ECT in anti-NMDAR encephalitis. Although it is true that ECT led to rapid and sometimes dramatic improvement, a lack of consistent reporting of improvement affects the interpretation. The absence of standardized assessment of response to treatment of anti-NMDAR encephalitis is a tremendous gap in the literature. The need for standardized methodology to assess outcomes in response to catatonia treatment was recognized in the 1990s with the development of the Bush Francis Catatonia Rating Scale (BFCRS).[33] Fourteen items were developed to screen for catatonia (BFCSI) with 9 additional items for assessment of severity (BFCRS). The BFCSI can help discriminate patients with catatonia from patients with other psychiatric presentations. Serial measurement using this scale enables clinicians to monitor response to treatment. There have also been other methods suggested in the literature for clinical monitoring including the clock drawing test.[34] The use of a standardized cognitive evaluation such as the Montreal Cognitive

Assessment (MoCA)[35] also needs to be explored; this tool has not been validated in children and adolescents except for a small study of adolescents with congenital heart disease.[36] Attempts have been made to develop an algorithm to guide treatment of autoimmune encephalitis.[37] However, the literature lacks integration of management of the immunologic aspects of the disease with management of the catatonic syndrome evident in the clinical symptoms.

Regardless of specific cause, use of BZDs and/or ECT for catatonia is indicated. Petrides and colleagues[38] identify BZD treatment as a safe and effective first-line treatment of catatonia. They identify the importance of a rapid shift to ECT when BZDs are thought to be ineffective. BFCRS was used to standardize assessment, and patients received either sequential treatment (BZDs and ECT) or concurrent treatment. The combined approach was superior to BZD treatment alone. When BZD was ineffective, ECT was added, and this resulted in improvement while the dose of BZDs either remained the same or was decreased. The results suggest ECT and BZDs are synergistic in efficacy.

We propose that a treatment algorithm for anti-NMDAR encephalitis should use both BZDs and/or ECT to manage catatonic symptoms in addition to immunotherapy to target the antibody development. ECT has been suggested to be particularly useful[35] in cases of resistant catatonia, failure of first-line immunotherapy, and unavailability of plasma exchanges. Based on the rapid improvement noted in the case reports, the use of synergistic ECT could also help with faster recovery and shorter time spent in the hospital.

Further research is needed to identify the treatment specifications such as length of time of treatment and parameters for response to treatment. Treatment progress should be measured by a validated tool such as BFCRS to document changes in severity of catatonia. It is also important to document changes in cognitive function. Tools such as the MoCA[35,36] or the Mini–Mental Status Examination[39] have been used but are not validated in the general child and adolescent population. Further consideration is needed to determine how to best monitor cognitive status. Future research should include development of a treatment algorithm that includes ECT as a potential component of disease management when the disease presentation includes the syndrome of catatonia.

REFERENCES

1. Dalmau J, Graus F. Antibody-mediated encephalitis. N Engl J Med 2018;378(9): 840–51.
2. Dalmau J, Tüzün E, Wu HY, et al. Paraneoplastic anti-N-methyl-D-aspartate receptor encephalitis associated with ovarian teratoma. Ann Neurol 2007;61(1): 25–36.
3. Dalmau J, Gleichman AJ, Hughes EG, et al. Anti-NMDA-receptor encephalitis: case series and analysis of the effects of antibodies. Lancet Neurol 2008;7(12): 1091–8.
4. Florance NR, Davis RL, Lam C, et al. Anti-N-methyl-D-aspartate receptor (NMDAR) encephalitis in children and adolescents. Ann Neurol 2009;66(1):11–8.
5. Titulaer MJ, McCracken L, Gabilondo I, et al. Treatment and prognostic factors for long-term outcome in patients with anti-NMDA receptor encephalitis: an observational cohort study. Lancet Neurol 2013;12(2):157–65.
6. Wandinger KP, Saschenbrecker S, Stoecker W, et al. Anti-NMDA-receptor encephalitis: a severe, multistage, treatable disorder presenting with psychosis. J Neuroimmunol 2011;231(1):86–91.

7. Irani SR, Bera K, Waters P, et al. N-methyl-D-aspartate antibody encephalitis: temporal progression of clinical and paraclinical observations in a predominantly non-paraneoplastic disorder of both sexes. Brain 2010;133(6):1655–67.

8. Coffey MJ, Cooper JJ. Electroconvulsive therapy in anti-N-Methyl-D-aspartate receptor encephalitis: a case report and review of the literature. J ECT 2016;32(4): 225–9.

9. Florance-Ryan N, Dalmau J. Update on anti-N-methyl-D-aspartate receptor encephalitis in children and adolescents. Curr Opin Pediatr 2010;22(6):739–44.

10. Wilson JE, Shuster J, Fuchs C. Anti-NMDA receptor encephalitis in a 14-year-old female presenting as malignant catatonia: medical and psychiatric approach to treatment. Psychosomatics 2013;54(6):585–9.

11. Diagnostic and statistical manual of mental disorders; revised (DSM-III-R). Washington, DC: American Psychiatric Association; 1987.

12. Pelzer AC, Van der Heijden FM, Den Boer E. Systematic review of catatonia treatment. Neuropsychiatr Dis Treat 2018;14:317.

13. Brar K, Kaushik SS, Lippmann S. Catatonia update. Prim Care Companion CNS Disord 2017;19(5) [pii:16br02023].

14. Diagnostic and statistical manual of mental disorders, text revision (DSM-IV-TR). Washington, DC: American Psychiatric Association; 2000.

15. Diagnostic and statistical manual of mental disorders (DSM-5®). Washington, DC: American Psychiatric Association; 2013.

16. Peter-Ross EM. Molecular hypotheses to explain the shared pathways and underlying pathobiological causes in catatonia and in catatonic presentations in neuropsychiatric disorders. Med Hypotheses 2018;113:54–64.

17. Morrison JR. Catatonia: diagnosis and management. Psychiatr Serv 1975;26(2): 91–4.

18. Rey JM, Walter G. Half a century of ECT use in young people. Am J Psychiatry 1997;154(5):595.

19. Fink M, Taylor MA. The catatonia syndrome: forgotten but not gone. Arch Gen Psychiatry 2009;66(11):1173–7.

20. Lesage A, Lemasson M, Medina K, et al. The prevalence of electroconvulsive therapy use since 1973: a meta-analysis. J ECT 2016;32(4):236–42.

21. Braakman HMH, Moers-Hornikx VMP, Arts BMG, et al. Pearls & oysters: electroconvulsive therapy in anti-NMDA receptor encephalitis. Neurology 2010;75(10): e44–6.

22. Matsumoto T, Matsumoto K, Kobayashi T, et al. Electroconvulsive therapy can improve psychotic symptoms in anti-NMDA-receptor encephalitis. Psychiatry Clin Neurosci 2012;66(3):242–3.

23. Mann A, Machado NM, Liu N, et al. A multidisciplinary approach to the treatment of anti-NMDA-receptor antibody encephalitis: a case and review of the literature. J Neuropsychiatry Clin Neurosci 2012;24(2):247–54.

24. Jones KC, Schwartz AC, Hermida AP, et al. A case of anti-NMDA receptor encephalitis treated with ECT. J Psychiatr Pract 2015;21(5):374–80.

25. Sunwoo JS, Jung DC, Choi JY, et al. Successful treatment of refractory dyskinesia secondary to anti-N-methyl-D-aspartate receptor encephalitis with electroconvulsive therapy. J ECT 2016;32(3):e13–4.

26. Lee A, Glick DB, Dinwiddie SH. Electroconvulsive therapy in a pediatric patient with malignant catatonia and paraneoplastic limbic encephalitis. J ECT 2006; 22(4):267–70.

27. Slooter AJ, Braun KP, Balk FJ, et al. Electroconvulsive therapy for malignant catatonia in childhood. Pediatr Neurol 2005;32(3):190–2.

28. Chamberlin P, Kotbi N, Sanchez-Barranco P, et al. Electroconvulsive therapy as an intervention for autoimmune neuropsychiatric disease. J ECT 2017;33(4): e44–5.

29. Singh A, Kar SK. How electroconvulsive therapy works?: understanding the neurobiological mechanisms. Clin Psychopharmacol Neurosci 2017;15(3):210.

30. Hoirisch-Clapauch S, Mezzasalma MA, Nardi AE. Pivotal role of tissue plasminogen activator in the mechanism of action of electroconvulsive therapy. J Psychopharmacol 2014;28(2):99–105.

31. Watkins CJ, Pei Q, Newberry NR. Differential effects of electroconvulsive shock on the glutamate receptor mRNAs for NR2A, NR2B and mGluR5b. Brain Res Mol Brain Res 1998;61(1–2):108–13.

32. McCall WV, Andrade C, Sienaert P. Searching for the mechanism (s) of ECT's therapeutic effect. J ECT 2014;30(2):87.

33. Bush G, Fink M, Petrides G, et al. Catatonia. I. Rating scale and standardized examination. Acta Psychiatr Scand 1996;93(2):129–36.

34. Medina M, Cooper JJ. Refractory catatonia due to N-methyl-D-aspartate receptor encephalitis responsive to electroconvulsive therapy: the clinical use of the clock drawing test. J ECT 2017;33(4):223–4.

35. Nasreddine ZS, Phillips NA, Bédirian V, et al. The montreal cognitive assessment, MoCA: a brief screening tool for mild cognitive impairment. J Am Geriatr Soc 2005;53(4):695–9.

36. Pike NA, Poulsen MK, Woo MA. Validity of the Montreal cognitive assessment screener in adolescents and young adults with and without congenital heart disease. Nurs Res 2017;66(3):222–30.

37. Ferrafiat V, Raffin M, Freri E, et al. A causality algorithm to guide diagnosis and treatment of catatonia due to autoimmune conditions in children and adolescents. Schizophr Res 2017. https://doi.org/10.1016/j.schres.2017.06.036.

38. Petrides G, Divadeenam KM, Bush G, et al. Synergism of lorazepam and electroconvulsive therapy in the treatment of catatonia. Biol Psychiatry 1997;42(5): 375–81.

39. Klein LE, Roca RP, McArthur J, et al. Univariate and multivariate analyses of the mental status examination. J Am Geriatr Soc 1985;33(7):483–8.

Electroconvulsive Therapy and Other Neuromodulation Techniques for the Treatment of Psychosis

Christopher Todd Maley, MD*, Jonathan Essary Becker, DO, MS, Elizabeth K.B. Shultz, DO

KEYWORDS

- Psychosis • First episode psychosis • Schizophrenia • Electroconvulsive therapy
- Transcranial magnetic therapy • Vagus nerve stimulation
- Transcranial direct current stimulation • Deep brain stimulation

KEY POINTS

- There is ample evidence supporting the use of electroconvulsive therapy (ECT) for the treatment of psychosis.
- ECT can be an effective add-on treatment for treatment-refractory patients already taking clozapine.
- Support for the use of ECT in patients experiencing a first episode of psychosis is growing.
- Parents of children who are provided with adequate information about ECT tend to have a more positive view of the procedure.
- Although there is some emerging evidence to support the use of alternative forms of neuromodulation (transcranial magnetic stimulation, transcranial direct current stimulation, vagus nerve stimulation, deep brain stimulation), none are currently supported for use in routine clinical management of psychosis.

INTRODUCTION

Schizophrenia was the initial indication for electroconvulsive therapy (ECT) in the 1930s when ECT was initially performed. However, the use of ECT for schizophrenia declined in the 1950s with the discovery of antipsychotic medications and increasing stigma with concerns for side effects.[1] Over the ensuing decades, the psychiatric community questioned the effectiveness of ECT for schizophrenia.[2] In 1978, the

Disclosure Statement: The authors have no disclosures to report.
Department of Psychiatry, Vanderbilt University Medical Center, Vanderbilt Psychiatric Hospital, 1601 23rd Avenue South, Nashville, TN 37212, USA
* Corresponding author.
E-mail address: christopher.maley@vanderbilt.edu

American Psychiatric Association Task Force for ECT stated that the data supporting or opposing the use of ECT for schizophrenia were inconclusive. Their ultimate recommendation was that ECT only be used for psychoses when there was an acute safety risk to the patient or others and when the patient could not be treated effectively with medications.[3] The second edition of the task force updated their recommendation in 2001 to recommend the use of ECT in schizophrenia when patients demonstrated an acute exacerbation of positive symptoms, had catatonic symptoms, had a history of past positive response to ECT, or had the presence of acute affective symptoms.[4] More recently, concerns with long-term side effects with the use of antipsychotics and the fact that 20% of patients are refractory to treatment with medications have led to a renewed interest and evaluation of the use of ECT.

ELECTROCONVULSIVE THERAPY FOR THE TREATMENT OF PSYCHOSIS

In a 2009 meta-analysis, Tharyan and Adams[1] reviewed the evidence for ECT in schizophrenia. They reviewed 10 articles, including 392 subjects that demonstrated that ECT was more effective than sham ECT with a number needed to treat of 6. All but 3 of the studies included in this analysis used comorbid treatment with antipsychotics in the active and sham ECT groups, which cloud the true effect of ECT because the efficacy of antipsychotics has been well established. One of the major benefits seen was that patients receiving active ECT demonstrated a much more rapid clinical global improvement than those who received sham treatment, especially when combined with antipsychotic medication. Considering the possible long-term benefits of ECT, Lin and colleagues[5] published a study analyzing data from claims records in Taiwan's National Health Insurance program. They found that, over the year following ECT, patients had fewer rehospitalizations, decreased emergency room visits, and lower overall health care costs than those who only received treatment with medications.

To assess the use of ECT in patients with treatment-refractory schizophrenia, Petrides and colleagues[6] conducted a randomized trial of patients receiving bilateral ECT plus clozapine versus patients receiving only clozapine. Subjects with affective symptoms were excluded. Of the subjects who received ECT plus clozapine, 50% met response criteria, as defined by a greater than 40% improvement in the psychotic symptoms subscale of the CGIs, whereas 0% in the clozapine-only group met response criteria. In a crossover phase, 47.4% of the subjects who did not meet response criteria in the randomized phase met response criteria in the crossover phase. These findings are quite impressive considering the utility of clozapine in the use of treatment-refractory schizophrenia. Grover and colleagues[7] further support the usefulness of ECT in refractory schizophrenia. They conducted a retrospective case review of 59 treatment-refractory schizophrenia patients on a combination of clozapine and ECT. They found that 60% of patients had a 30% reduction in Positive and Negative Syndrome Scale (PANSS). Impressively, long-term follow-up was available for 47 of the 59 after 1 year, and 72% of these patients had maintained their response, highlighting the durability of ECT for refractory schizophrenia.

Relapse prevention in schizophrenia is another clinical challenge. In mood disorders, maintenance ECT can be an effective treatment modality to maintain response to treatment. The idea of maintenance ECT in schizophrenia was recently reviewed by Ward and colleagues.[8] They reviewed 118 articles and ultimately included 37 studies in their analysis. Only 2 of these were randomized controlled trials. In the randomized controlled trials, Chanpattana and colleagues[9] found relapse rates of 40% with a combination of ECT and flupentixol versus 93% for both medication-only and maintenance ECT–only groups. Yang and colleagues[10] showed that those receiving ECT plus risperidone were statistically significantly less likely to relapse over 12 months than those receiving risperidone only. In evaluation of the other 35 studies, Ward and colleagues concluded that the available evidence showed that patients that receive maintenance ECT demonstrate sustained improvement.

The major concern many clinicians and patients have regarding ECT is cognitive impairment. Schizophrenia is also associated with cognitive impairment raising further concern for the use of ECT in schizophrenia. To assess the effects of ECT on cognition, Cusa and colleagues[11] conducted a recent study in 2018. They sampled 31 inpatients diagnosed with treatment-resistant schizophrenia. The effects of ECT were examined using a battery of neuropsychological tests administered 1 day before ECT and 1 day after ECT applications. In addition to finding that patients who received ECT exhibited less clinical symptoms, they also found statistically significant improvement in immediate and delayed total recall and the Stroop Interference test, which measures executive functioning and cognitive flexibility. They also found statistical trends for improvement in the Stroop Color-Block test, which measures psychomotor speed and visual memory. The remainder of the neurocognitive functioning showed no difference pre-ECT and post-ECT but did not worsen for the ECT group. Tor and colleagues[12] also provide evidence that ECT may improve cognitive performance in ECT. They found an improvement of MoCA scores after ECT with an overall mean improvement from 16.8 pre-ECT to 20.7 post-ECT.

Electroconvulsive Therapy and First Episode Psychosis

ECT has long been established as an effective treatment for various psychiatric illnesses in adults, particularly mood disorders and catatonia. In more recent years, there has been growing evidence and support for treating adolescents with mood disorders and catatonia using ECT as well. In fact, in 2004, the American Academy of Child and Adolescent Psychiatry released its parameters for the use of ECT in adolescents. Most recently, the use of ECT in the treatment of psychotic disorders, especially first episode psychosis, is gaining support as evidenced by recent publications in the international community, including case reports and clinical trials. For reference in this discussion, intractable or treatment-resistant psychosis means failure of an adequate (at least 4 weeks) trial of at least 2 antipsychotics or intolerability of antipsychotics due to side effects.

In 2006, results from a prospective study examined "short-term effects of acute ECT and its safety in young adults with medically intractable first-episode schizophrenia."[13] The investigators examined 7 patients with first episode schizophrenia or schizophreniform disorder resistant to treatment with medications alone. Measures for progress were the Brief Psychiatric Rating Scale and Global Assessment of Functioning (GAF) scores, both of which improved significantly in each patient after a course of ECT. "Mild delirium"[13] was the only adverse event reported; thus, the investigators concluded that ECT could be a safe and effective treatment of treatment-resistant first episode psychosis.

In 2015, a published case report of a 10-year-old male child presenting with acute psychosis and catatonic symptoms detailed the use of ECT in managing his illness.[14] He received a combination of injections of lorazepam, oral olanzapine, and 5 treatments of bilateral ECT to induce resolution of his symptoms. No adverse effects were reported in this case.

A series of publications from investigators at the Hospital Clinic of Barcelona's Neurosciences Institute Clinic examined several aspects of ECT use in adolescents, including ECT combined with clozapine, the opinions of parents of adolescents with schizophrenia spectrum disorders treated with ECT, short-term and long-term efficacy of ECT in adolescents with schizophrenia spectrum disorders, and cognitive effects of ECT use in adolescents. Each article is discussed individually in later discussion.

Clozapine is known to be one of the most effective antipsychotics available, particularly in patients who have not responded to other agents. Investigators at the Hospital Clinic of Barcelona examined whether the combination of ECT and clozapine yielded any increase in adverse effects or change in rate of rehospitalization compared with a matched group treated with ECT and other antipsychotics or benzodiazepines.[15] Twenty-eight adolescents diagnosed with treatment-resistant schizophrenia spectrum disorders were compared (16 had been treated with ECT and other antipsychotics or benzodiazepines, whereas the remaining 12 were treated with ECT and clozapine). Equivalent safety was observed in both groups, and both groups received effective treatment; however, the ECT plus clozapine group had fewer instances of repeat hospitalizations at follow-up 1 year later.

It is commonly thought that negative stigma about ECT increases resistance to considering or accepting ECT as a treatment. This stigma may be perceived by treating physicians, patients, or families of patients. In a 2017 publication, the investigators examined the opinions of parents whose child received ECT as a treatment for schizophrenia spectrum disorder versus parents whose child did not receive this treatment.[16] In addition, the investigators explored the experience of the parents whose children received ECT by asking opinions on the amount of information provided about the treatment modality, on safety of the treatment, and on efficacy of the treatment. Generally, the parents whose children received ECT thought the treatment was safe and that they had received appropriate amounts of information about the treatment, and the majority thought the treatment had been helpful for the child. In contrast, a significantly lower proportion of the parents of children who received only medication thought they had adequate knowledge about ECT and whether it is a safe and effective treatment. Parents in both groups responded that they would agree to ECT if recommended for their children in the future. The most significant difference between the 2 groups of parents appeared to be the knowledge gap regarding information about ECT, which in turn influenced the opinion as to whether ECT was a safe and effective treatment. Of note, because this study was conducted in Spain, there may be regional or other factors that may not be generalizable to populations elsewhere, and replication of these results elsewhere would be an important future direction.

Two separate publications examined the efficacy of ECT in adolescents with schizophrenia spectrum disorders, one looking at more immediate results and one looking at longer-term results. A third publication examined the cognitive functions of adolescents with schizophrenia spectrum disorders treated with ECT at 2-years post-ECT. These publications are discussed later.

In the 2010 publication, the investigators retrospectively reviewed patients diagnosed with schizophrenia spectrum disorders who received ECT and assessed efficacy of the treatment based on PANSS scores (positive, negative, general, and total) and Clinical Global Impression (CGI) scales pre-ECT and at 6 months post-ECT.[17] Side effects were also noted. A total of 13 patients met the inclusion criteria and received "constant-current, brief pulse" bifrontotemporal treatments. There was significant improvement in the PANSS positive, general, and total scores; however, there was no significant change in the PANSS negative scores. CGI ratings also improved significantly. No serious adverse effects were reported, suggesting the safety of the treatment performed.

Later, in 2011, a different group of investigators from the same institution as the 2010 publication examined the cognitive function of adolescents who received ECT as treatment of schizophrenia spectrum disorders at 2-years posttreatment.[18] They examined cognitive function in 9 adolescents who received ECT as treatment and compared them with a matched group of 9 adolescents who did not receive ECT. Neuropsychological testing was administered to each group at baseline and again at 2 years; moreover, PANSS and CGI scales were administered at the same intervals. Both groups showed significant improvement in PANSS (positive, general, total, but not negative) and CGI ratings as well as significant improvement in cognitive performance on verbal fluency and digits forward tasks. There was no significant difference between the 2 groups at follow-up, suggesting that ECT did not lead to any negative long-term effects cognitively.

Finally, in a 2015 publication from the same institution, long-term follow-up comparisons between an ECT group and a matched non-ECT (medication only) group were examined. Each patient was rated on the PANSS, CGI, and GAF at baseline and follow-up. Notable differences between the groups include that the ECT group generally was younger at age of onset, had had more medication failures, and initially had significantly different CGI, GAF, and PANSS total, negative, and general scores (high scores) in the ECT group, yet there was no significant difference between the groups in the PANSS negative scores.[19] Both groups exhibited significant improvements in CGI, GAF, and PANSS positive, general, and total scores at follow-up, whereas neither group had a significant difference in PANSS negative scores. The ECT patients had fewer hospitalizations and required fewer antipsychotics after ECT than before this treatment. CGI and GAF did not significantly differ between the groups at follow-up; PANSS total, general, and positive were significantly higher in the ECT group than the non-ECT group at follow-up. Although there were significant differences between the severity of symptoms of each group at follow-up, overall, there was improvement from baseline in both groups. These results suggest that ECT can have long-term effectiveness in treating adolescents with schizophrenia spectrum disorders.

Collectively, these publications help build a case that ECT can be a safe, effective treatment in first episode psychosis, such as schizophrenia spectrum disorders, particularly in treatment-resistant patients.

OTHER NEUROMODULATION APPROACHES FOR THE TREATMENT OF PSYCHOSIS
Transcranial Magnetic Stimulation

Transcranial Magnetic Stimulation (TMS) is a noninvasive treatment technique in which repetitive magnetic field pulses are delivered from a coil through the scalp, stimulating brain tissue underneath. TMS was approved for the treatment of major depressive disorder as defined in the *Diagnostic and Statistical Manual of Mental Disorders* (fourth edition) and has also been studied for the off-label treatment of several other psychiatric conditions, including psychotic disorders such as schizophrenia. TMS has also been used to evaluate and treat neurologic conditions in childhood such as epilepsy, headache, perinatal stroke, and cerebral palsy.[20]

Investigations into the utility of TMS for schizophrenia in adults have generally focused on treatment of positive (hallucinations, primarily) and negative (avolition, apathy, cognitive dulling) symptoms. Most studies examining positive symptoms have looked at low-frequency (1 Hz) TMS targeting the left temporoparietal cortex (TPC).[21–23] For negative symptoms, several studies have investigated higher-frequency TMS applied to the dorsolateral prefrontal cortex.[24–26]

Research regarding the use of TMS for the treatment of schizophrenia in children and adolescents is admittedly limited. In 2007, Jardri and colleagues[27] described the successful treatment of an 11-year-old boy with low-frequency (1 Hz) TMS applied to the left TPC; they later described the successful and sustained treatment of auditory hallucinations within a cohort of adolescents using the same technique. Several other case studies have described similar findings.[28–30] To date, there have been no large clinical trials investigating the use of TMS as a first-line treatment for the treatment of childhood-onset schizophrenia.

TMS is a generally well-tolerated procedure and is thought to be safe for use in children, and there are few absolute or relative contraindications to its use, examples of which are ferromagnetic material in the head, intracardiac lines, increased intracranial pressure, and cochlear implants (absolute); and cardiac pacemakers, implanted medication pumps, ventriculoperitoneal shunts, and some medications, including antipsychotics, antidepressants, antianxiety medications, and tricyclics (relative).[31]

Deep Brain Stimulation

Deep brain stimulation (DBS) involves a neurosurgical procedure in which electrodes are implanted into target brain structures and connected to a battery that is implanted in the chest. Once the device is activated, it delivers electrical impulses directly into the targets. DBS carries US Food and Drug Administration approval for the treatment of movement disorders, medically refractory epilepsy, and a sole psychiatric disorder, obsessive compulsive disorder (OCD). It has been used as an investigative tool for the treatment of several other psychiatric conditions, however, including major depressive disorder, anorexia nervosa, and posttraumatic stress disorder.[32]

Regarding schizophrenia, DBS is theorized to have potential benefit by targeting specific brain structures, such as the anterior hippocampus (to reduce dopaminergic hyperactivity) and the nucleus accumbens (by balancing dopaminergic balance).[33,34] DBS may also help normalize neural oscillations, disruptions of which may contribute to cognitive and attentional deficits commonly seen in schizophrenia.[33] A limited number of phase I clinical DBS trials have shown initial improvement in both positive and negative symptoms.[35] DBS is generally well tolerated, although serious complications can occur, including intracerebral hemorrhage and infection.[36] In the study of Saleh and Fontaine[37] of 272 patients who received DBS for psychiatric conditions (OCD, Tourette syndrome, treatment-resistant depression), the most common adverse events were mood alterations, hardware-related complications, and anxiety. Interestingly, psychosis was noted as a complication in 1.5% of patients.

Transcranial Direct Current Stimulation

Transcranial direct current stimulation (tDCS) is a treatment modality in which a weak current of electricity is passed through electrodes from the scalp to the brain. The current is sufficient to stimulate neuronal activity but is not sufficient to produce depolarizing action potentials. tDCS has a more favorable side-effect profile versus TMS and has been studied for the treatment of several neurologic and psychiatric conditions in children and adolescents, including epilepsy, dystonias, attention-deficit/hyperactivity disorder, autism spectrum disorder, and childhood-onset schizophrenia.[38]

The adult literature suggests that tDCS may be helpful in the treatment of multiple symptom domains in schizophrenia (reduction in negative symptoms by anodal stimulation of the left dorsolateral prefrontal cortex and improvement in auditory hallucinations by the cathodal inhibitory stimulation of the left temporoparietal junction).[39] In addition, a 2017 review by Mervis and colleagues[40] suggests that both anodal and cathodal stimulation may mitigate deficits of attention, working memory, and cognitive abilities in the disorder. Other studies, however, are less promising and have either failed to show an effect[41] or have not shown superiority to placebo.[42] A 2011 study by Mattai and colleagues[43] showed that tDCS was well tolerated in the pediatric population with itching, tingling, and fatigue being the most commonly reported side effects.[43] Studies involving the treatment of children and adolescents with tDCS for schizophrenia are admittedly limited.

Vagal Nerve Stimulation

Vagal nerve stimulation (VNS) is a treatment modality in which the brain is stimulated indirectly by electrical impulses passed along the vagus nerve (the tenth cranial nerve) emitted by a generator that is either surgically implanted or is noninvasive (transcutaneous vagal nerve stimulation, or tVNS). VNS is approved in the United States for the treatment of epilepsy and treatment-resistant depression. VNS is approved for the treatment of epilepsy in children as young as 4, but presently there are no indications for use in child or adolescent psychiatric conditions.

Studies using VNS for the treatment of schizophrenia-associated symptoms are quite limited. A 2015 study by Hasan and colleagues[44] looked at tVNS for the treatment of schizophrenia; this was a randomized, double-blind study in which 20 patients received either active or sham treatment. Although the treatment itself was well tolerated, outcomes were not statistically significant between the 2 groups. Perez and colleagues[45] have looked at the use of VNS in a rodent model of schizophrenia (methylazoxymethanol acetate model); in their 2014 study, VNS was targeted toward the ventral hippocampus and demonstrated a reversal of hyperactivity in this area as well as in the mesolimbic dopaminergic pathway. Rats treated with VNS in the study showed a lack of locomotor response to a dose of amphetamine when compared with the control group. VNS may also show utility for the treatment of schizophrenia through cognitive-enhancing effects, increasing cholinergic neurotransmission, and increasing serotonin release.[46]

Interestingly, there is some evidence to suggest that VNS may precipitate or contribute to psychiatric pathologic condition in patients with preexisting epilepsy.[47,48] Blumer and colleagues[47] looked at 81 patients treated with VNS for 6 months; 7 patients developed significant psychiatric complications, including psychosis, dysphoria, or a combination of the 2. Vagus nerve stimulation is a generally well-tolerated procedure. A small number of patients may experience stimulation-related side effects, such as hoarseness and dysphagia.[49] Although rare, more serious complications include postoperative hematoma and infection.[49,50]

SUMMARY

ECT is an established treatment for symptoms of psychosis and is currently recommended for use in patients who are experiencing an acute exacerbation of positive symptoms or who have had catatonia. There is also evidence to suggest that ECT can be a safe, effective treatment in first episode psychosis, such as schizophrenia spectrum disorders, particularly in treatment-resistant patients. Other forms of neuromodulation (TMS, tDCS, VNS, DBS) have less of an evidence base to support their use and are not formally indicated for the treatment of psychosis.

REFERENCES

1. Tharyan P, Adams CE. Electroconvulsive therapy for schizophrenia. Cochrane Database Syst Rev 2005;(2):CD000076.

2. Fink M, Sackeim HA. Convulsive therapy for schizophrenia? Schizophr Bull 1996; 22(1):29–39.
3. American Psychiatric Association. Report of the task force on electroconvulsive therapy of the American Psychiatric Association. Washington, DC: American Psychiatric Association; 1978.
4. American Psychiatric Association. Committee on electroconvulsive therapy. The practice of electroconvulsive therapy: recommendations for treatment, training, and privileging: a task force report of the American Psychiatric Association. 2nd edition. Washington, DC: American Psychiatric Association; 2001.
5. Lin H, Liu S, Hsieh MH, et al. Impacts of electroconvulsive therapy on 1-year outcomes in patients with schizophrenia: a controlled, population-based mirror-image study. Schizophr Bull 2017. https://doi.org/10.1093/schbul/sbx136.
6. Petrides G, Malur C, Braga R, et al. Electroconvulsive therapy augmentation in clozapine-resistant schizophrenia: a prospective, randomized study. Am J Psychiatry 2015;172(1):52–8.
7. Grover S, Chakrabarti S, Hazari N, et al. Effectiveness of electroconvulsive therapy in patients with treatment resistant schizophrenia: a retrospective study. Psychiatry Res 2017;249:349–53.
8. Ward HB, Szabo ST, Rakesh G. Maintenance ECT in schizophrenia: a systematic review. Psychiatry Res 2018;264:131–42.
9. Chanpattana W, Chakrabhand MS, Sackeim HA, et al. Continuation ECT in treatment-resistant schizophrenia: a controlled study. J ECT 1999;15(3):178–92.
10. Yang Y, Cheng X, Xu Q, et al. The maintenance of modified electroconvulsive therapy combined with risperidone is better than risperidone alone in preventing relapse of schizophrenia and improving cognitive function. Arq Neuropsiquiatr 2016;74(10):823–8.
11. Cusa VK, Klepac N, Jaksic N, et al. The effects of electroconvulsive therapy augmentation of antipsychotic treatment on cognitive functions in patients with treatment-resistant schizophrenia. J ECT 2018;34(1):31–4.
12. Tor PC, Ying J, Ho NF, et al. Effectiveness of electroconvulsive therapy and associated cognitive change in schizophrenia: a naturalistic, comparative study of treating schizophrenia with electroconvulsive therapy. J ECT 2017;33:272–7.
13. Suzuki K, Awata S, Takano T, et al. Improvement of psychiatric symptoms after electroconvulsive therapy in young adults with intractable first-episode schizophrenia and schizophreniform disorder. Tohoku J Exp Med 2006;210(3):213–20.
14. Mohapatra S, Rath N. Electroconvulsive therapy in a child suffering from acute and transient psychotic disorder with catatonic features. Indian J Psychol Med 2015;37:465–6.
15. Flamarique I, Castro-Fornieles J, Garrido JM, et al. Electroconvulsive therapy and clozapine in adolescents with schizophrenia spectrum disorders: is it a safe and effective combination? J Clin Psychopharmacol 2012;32(6):756–66.
16. Flamarique I, Baeza I, de la Serna E, et al. Thinking about electroconvulsive therapy: the opinions of parents of adolescents with schizophrenia spectrum disorders. J Child Adolesc Psychopharmacol 2017;27(1):75–82.
17. Baeza I, Flamarique I, Garrido JM, et al. Clinical experience using electroconvulsive therapy in adolescents with schizophrenia spectrum disorders. J Child Adolesc Psychopharmacol 2010;20(3):205–9.
18. De la Serna E, Flamarique I, Castro-Fornieles J, et al. Two year follow up of cognitive functions in schizophrenia spectrum disorders of adolescent patients treated with electroconvulsive therapy. J Child Adolesc Psychopharmacol 2011. https://doi.org/10.1089/cap2011.0012.

19. Flamarique I, Baeza I, de la Serna E, et al. Long-term effectiveness of electrocon-vulsive therapy in adolescents with schizophrenia spectrum disorders. Eur Child Adolesc Psychiatry 2015;24:517.
20. Rajapakse T, Kirton A. Non-invasive brain stimulation in children: applications and future directions. Transl Neurosci 2013;4(2):1–29.
21. Freitas C, Fregni F, Pascual-Leone A. Meta-analysis of the effects of repetitive transcranial magnetic stimulation (rTMS) on negative and positive symptoms in schizophrenia. Schizophr Res 2009;108:11–24.
22. Nieuwdorp W, Koops S, Somers M, et al. Transcranial magnetic stimulation, trans-cranial direct current stimulation and electroconvulsive therapy for medication-resistant psychosis of schizophrenia. Curr Opin Psychiatry 2015;28:222–8.
23. Slotema C, Blom J, van Lutterveld R, et al. Review of the efficacy of transcranial magnetic stimulation for auditory verbal hallucinations. Biol Psychiatry 2014;76:101–10.
24. Dlabac-de Lange J, Knegtering R, Aleman A. Repetitive transcranial magnetic stimulation for negative symptoms of schizophrenia: review and meta-analysis. J Clin Psychiatry 2010;71(4):411–8.
25. Shi C, Yu X, Cheung E, et al. Revisiting the therapeutic effect of rTMS on negative symptoms in schizophrenia: a meta-analysis. Psychiatry Res 2014; 215:505–13.
26. Prikryl R, Kucerova H. Can repetitive transcranial magnetic stimulation be consid-ered effective treatment option for negative symptoms of schizophrenia? J ECT 2013;29:67–74.
27. Jardri R, Lucas B, Delevoye-Turrell Y, et al. An 11-year-old boy with drug-resistant schizophrenia treated with temporo-parietal rTMS. Mol Psychiatry 2007;12(4):320.
28. Walter G, Tormos JM, Israel JA, et al. Transcranial magnetic stimulation in young persons: a review of known cases. J Child Adolesc Psychopharmacol 2001;11(1):69–75.
29. Fitzgerald PB, Benitez J, Daskalakis JZ, et al. The treatment of recurring auditory hallucinations in schizophrenia with rTMS. World J Biol Psychiatry 2006;7(2):119–22.
30. Hoffman RE, Hawkins KA, Gueorguieva R, et al. Transcranial magnetic stimula-tion of left temporoparietal cortex and medication-resistant auditory hallucina-tions. Arch Gen Psychiatry 2003;60(1):49–56.
31. Narayana S, Papanicolaou AC, McGregor A, et al. Clinical applications of trans-cranial magnetic stimulation in pediatric neurology. J Child Neurol 2015;30(9):1111–24.
32. Cleary D, Ozpinar A, Raslan A, et al. Deep brain stimulation for psychiatric disor-ders: where we are now. Neurosurg Focus 2015;38(6):E2, 1-24.
33. Kuhn J, Bodatsch M, Sturm V, et al. Deep brain stimulation in schizophrenia. Act Nerv Super 2014;56(3):69–78.
34. Mikell C, McKhann G, Segal S, et al. The hippocampus and nucleus accumbens as potential therapeutic targets for neurosurgical intervention in schizophrenia. Stereotact Funct Neurosurg 2009;87:256–65.
35. Gault JM, Davis R, Cascella NG, et al. Approaches to neuromodulation for schizophrenia. J Neurol Neurosurg Psychiatry 2018;89(7):777–87.
36. Schermer M. Ethical issues in deep brain stimulation. Front Integr Neurosci 2011;5:1–5.
37. Saleh C, Fontaine D. Deep brain stimulation for psychiatric diseases: what are the risks? Curr Psychiatry Rep 2015;17(5):33.

38. Palm U, Segmiller F, Epple A, et al. Transcranial direct current stimulation in children and adolescents: a comprehensive review. J Neural Transm 2016;123: 1219–34.

39. Brunelin J, Mondino M, Gassab L, et al. Examining transcranial direct-current stimulation (tDCS) as a treatment for hallucinations in schizophrenia. Am J Psychiatry 2012;169:719–24.

40. Mervis J, Capizzi R, Boroda E, et al. Transcranial direct current stimulation over the dorsolateral prefrontal cortex in schizophrenia: a quantitative review of cognitive outcomes. Front Hum Neurosci 2017;11:44, 1-8.

41. Fitzgerald PB, McQueen S, Daskalakis ZJ, et al. A negative pilot study of daily bimodal transcranial direct current stimulation in schizophrenia. Brain Stimul 2014;7(6):813–6.

42. Fröhlich F, Burrello TN, Mellin JM, et al. Exploratory study of once-daily transcranial direct current stimulation (tDCS) as a treatment for auditory hallucinations in schizophrenia. Eur Psychiatry 2016;33:54–60.

43. Mattai A, Miller R, Weisinger B, et al. Tolerability of transcranial direct current stimulation in childhood-onset schizophrenia. Brain Stimul 2011;4:275–80.

44. Hasan A, Wolff-Menzler C, Pfeiffer S, et al. Transcutaneous noninvasive vagus nerve stimulation (tVNS) in the treatment of schizophrenia: a bicentric randomized controlled pilot study. Eur Arch Psychiatry Clin Neurosci 2015;265(7): 589–600.

45. Perez S, Carreno F, Frazer A, et al. Vagal nerve stimulation reverses aberrant dopamine system function in the Methylazoxymethanol acetate rodent model of schizophrenia. J Neurosci 2014;34(28):9261–7.

46. Smucny J, Visani A, Tregellas J. Could vagus nerve stimulation target hippocampal hyperactivity to improve cognition in schizophrenia. Front Psychiatry 2015;6: 1–5.

47. Blumer D, Davies K, Alexander A, et al. Major psychiatric disorders subsequent to treating epilepsy by vagus nerve stimulation. Epilepsy Behav 2001;2:466–72.

48. Keller S, Lichtenberg P. Psychotic exacerbation in a patient with seizure disorder treated with vagus nerve stimulation. Isr Med Assoc J 2008;10:550–1.

49. Smyth MD, Tubbs RS, Bebin EM, et al. Complications of chronic vagus nerve stimulation for epilepsy in children. J Neurosurg 2003;99:500–3.

50. Revesz D, Rydenhag B, Ben-Menachem E. Complications and safety of vagus nerve stimulation: 25 years of experience at a single center 2016;18:97–104.

Electroconvulsive Treatment for Catatonia in Autism Spectrum Disorders

Nisha Withane, MD[a], Dirk M. Dhossche, MD, PhD[b],*

KEYWORDS

- Catatonia • Autism spectrum disorder • Electroconvulsive treatment (ECT)
- Benzodiazepines

KEY POINTS

- Catatonia has been increasingly recognized as a comorbid syndrome of autism at a rate of 12% to 17% in adolescents and young adults with autism spectrum disorders.
- Upsetting life events, the loss of routine and structure, experiences of loss, conflicts with parents, caregivers, or peers, and discrepancies between the ability in the patient and parental expectations, especially, in higher functioning autistic youth, are known to precipitate catatonia.
- Lacking controlled trials, successful use of benzodiazepines and electroconvulsive treatment (ECT) for catatonia in autism is supported by case reports and case series.
- ECT is indicated for the treatment of catatonia when lorazepam does not bring about rapid relief. Maintenance ECT is important for sustained symptom remission.
- Preliminary reports support safety and tolerability of maintenance ECT in autistic patients who show stable neuropsychological testing during treatment.

INTRODUCTION

Catatonia has been increasingly recognized as a comorbid syndrome of autism spectrum disorders (ASD) in adolescents and young adults with ASD[1,2] and with other intellectual disabilities.[3,4] Two systematic clinician-based studies show that catatonia is found in 12% to 17% of adolescents and young adults with autism.[1,2]

Wing and Shah[2] reported that 17% of a large referred sample of adolescents and young adults with autism satisfied modern criteria for catatonia. Thirty individuals with autism aged 15 years or older met criteria for catatonia, with classic autistic disorder diagnosed in 11 (37%), atypical autism in 5 (17%), and Asperger disorder in 14

Disclosure Statement: The authors have no conflicts of interest.
[a] Department of Psychiatry, Institute of Living/Hartford Hospital, 200 Retreat Avenue, Hartford, CT 06106, USA; [b] Department of Psychiatry, University of Mississippi Medical Center, 2500 North State Street, Jackson, MS 39216, USA
* Corresponding author.
E-mail address: dirkdhossche@gmail.com

Child Adolesc Psychiatric Clin N Am 28 (2019) 101–110
https://doi.org/10.1016/j.chc.2018.07.006
1056-4993/19/© 2018 Elsevier Inc. All rights reserved.

(47%). Under age 15, no child demonstrated the full syndrome, although isolated catatonic symptoms were often observed. In most cases, catatonic symptoms started between 10 and 19 years of age. Five individuals had brief episodes of slowness and freezing during childhood before age 10. Obsessive-compulsive and aggressive behaviors preceded catatonia in some cases. Visual hallucinations or paranoid ideas were occasionally reported, but no diagnosis of schizophrenia could be made.

In the second study, 13 (12%) of 120 autistic individuals, between ages 17 and 40 years, had clinically diagnosed catatonia with severe motor initiation problems.[1] Another 4 individuals had several catatonic symptoms but did not meet criteria for the full syndrome. Eight of the 13 individuals with catatonia suffered from autistic disorder; the remaining 5 were diagnosed with atypical autism. The proportion of those with autistic disorder that were diagnosed with catatonia was 11% (8/73). Fourteen percent (5/35) of those with atypical autism had catatonia.

A hospital-based study[5] of 101 child and adolescent psychiatric inpatients with "at-risk" diagnoses, including any pervasive developmental disorder, psychotic disorder not otherwise specified, intermittent explosive disorder, intellectual developmental disorder, neuroleptic malignant syndrome, or previously diagnosed catatonia, found that 18% of patients met criteria for catatonia, based on 3 or more symptoms, including unexplained agitation or excitement, disturbed or unusual movements, reduction in movement, reduction or loss of speech, and repetitive/stereotyped movements. The investigators emphasized poor recognition of catatonia in these pediatric conditions, including, but not limited to, pervasive development disorders.

Breen and Hare[6] developed a 34-item third-party report measure, the Attenuated Behaviour Questionnaire (ABQ), consisting of 15 motor symptoms, 5 affective alterations, and 14 behavioral alterations, commonly associated with catatonia in ASD. They tested the new measure in a British sample of convenience (N = 99) of young people aged 12 to 25 years with existing diagnosis of ASD by interviewing the parent or long-term caregiver. Full data were available from 87 informants, of whom 18 (21%) reported an existing diagnosis of catatonia. Forty-two (48%) cases displayed 3 of more core catatonia-like attenuated behaviors. Scores on this new measure ABQ were higher in those with an existing catatonia diagnosis. Catatonia-like attenuated behaviors were associated with measures of depression and repetitive and restricted behaviors. The study did not report on how the existing clinical diagnoses of catatonia (as reported by parents or caregivers) were established but supports the ABQ as a clinical and research tool for catatonia symptoms in an ASD population.

In another study,[7] the same measure was completed by parents or caregivers of 33 individuals with Cornelia de Lange syndrome and 69 individuals with fragile X syndrome. Thirty percent of those with Cornelia de Lange syndrome and 12% of those with fragile X syndrome scored above the cutoff for catatonia-like attenuated behavior, supporting the presence of a catatonia-like syndrome in a significant number of people with these genetic syndromes. The study did assess the subjects directly or by clinical examinations, thereby precluding a comparison between those with and without clinical diagnoses of catatonia and precluding correlations between clinical diagnoses and ABQ scores by parents/caregivers.

Catatonia is often viewed as an epiphenomenon of another syndrome, such as depression,[8] bipolar illness,[9] or schizophrenia,[10] yet many patients with ASD cannot be diagnosed with a definite affective or psychotic disorder due to the fact that these patients are nonverbal and have severe cognitive impairments.

Case reports also describe catatonia in pediatric patients with Prader-Willi syndrome[3] and Down syndrome,[11] genetic disorders that are characterized by varying degrees of developmental impairment, autistic features, and medical and behavioral abnormalities that are specific to the genetic defect.

Most cases of catatonia in children and adolescents with ASD are not associated with any underlying clearly identifiable medical or psychiatric conditions. For example, in a sample of 58 children and adolescents with catatonia,[12] 18 (31%) had a history of developmental disorder, that is, ASD, intellectual disability, or neurodevelopmental malformation. Only 2 of those had an identifiable underlying medical or psychiatric condition.

SYMPTOMS OF CATATONIA IN AUTISM SPECTRUM DISORDERS

Catatonia in ASD is currently diagnosed in *Diagnostic and Statistical Manual of Mental Disorders* (Fifth Edition) based on the presence of 3 out of 12 symptoms[13]: catalepsy, waxy flexibility, stupor, agitation, mutism, negativism, posturing, mannerisms, stereotypies, grimacing, echolalia, or echopraxia. These symptoms may be present at baseline in patients with ASD but a low severity and with low frequency without much functional impairment. However, a sharp increase of these preexisting symptoms or sudden appearance of new catatonic symptoms should alert the clinician to assess for a diagnosis of catatonia.[2,14,15]

Several catatonia rating scales have been developed.[16] The most commonly used scale for the assessment of catatonia is the Bush-Francis Catatonia Scale (BFCRS),[17] a 23-item standardized instrument that is designed for diagnosing and for the assessment of severity. When using the BFCRS, catatonia may be diagnosed when 2 or more items on the first 17 items are present. Serial catatonia ratings are useful to detail changes over time and for measuring change during treatment[18] in individual cases and controlled studies. Although the BFCRS is useful in patients with autism, the scale was developed using a sample of general adult psychiatric patients. There are currently no catatonia rating scales that have been standardized in patients with autism. The KANNER scale, named after Leo Kanner (1894–1981) who described the neuromotor and neurodevelopmental features of autism,[19] has been proposed as a unifying instrument for quantifying core features of catatonia, across a broad range of neuropsychiatric disorders, including autism and pervasive developmental disorders.[20] The scale is comprehensive; however, it is untested and not validated in patients with autism.

As described earlier, the 34-item third-party report ABQ has been developed based on behaviors and symptoms commonly associated with catatonia in ASD.[6] The scale consists of 15 motor symptoms, 5 affective alterations, and 14 behavioral features. The scale is supported as a clinical and research tool for catatonia symptoms in an ASD population[6] and in other samples of patients with developmental disorder[7] but requires further testing and validation in samples with concurrent clinical assessments.

Self-injurious behavior (SIB) occurs regularly in patients with ASD and includes behaviors such as self-hitting, punching, biting, scratching, and kicking. SIB can lead to significant injury to soft tissue, bone, head trauma, retinal detachment, blindness, or even death.[21] Often SIB is under operant conditioning[22]; however, sudden increases of SIB may sometimes be a part of the constellation of stereotypical behaviors seen in catatonia. Wing and Shah[23] reported the presence of catatonic stereotypies in 23% to 46% of autistic patients they assessed. Although they did not assess self-injury as a stereotypical behavior, however, the repetitive nature of these behaviors suggests that there is a significant correlation between SIB, catatonia, and ASD. Wachtel and Dhossche[24] hypothesized that some patients with ASD featuring extreme levels or increases of SIB could suffer from underlying catatonia and should be assessed for other symptoms of catatonia, and, as such, could be treated with electroconvulsive treatment (ECT). The initial and promising experiences in this area and the positive effects of ECT in such cases have been described elsewhere.[25]

BENZODIAZEPINES AND ELECTROCONVULSIVE TREATMENT ARE THE EMPIRICAL TREATMENTS OF CHOICE FOR CATATONIA IN AUTISM SPECTRUM DISORDERS

In 2014, DeJong and colleagues[26] reviewed all pertinent papers from 1980 onwards on interventions used to treat catatonia in ASD, identifying 22 relevant papers on 28 cases both adult and pediatric, with the majority coming from the United States. They report some support for the use of ECT, high-dose lorazepam, and behavioral interventions in this patient group and lament the lack of strong evidence in this field, small number of cases, an evidence base consisting entirely of case studies, small case series, and clinical opinion, poor quality in terms of treatment protocols, and objective measures of outcome. The study emphasizes the urgent need for prospective long-term studies and controlled trials.

Case Vignette 1

X is a 16-year-old male patient with ASD and severe intellectual disability who presented to the hospital after his outpatient neurologist had concerns for significant changes in his behavior and his inability to take care of his activities of daily living (ADLs; bathing, feeding, dressing, and his ability to use the bathroom on his own). At his baseline, X was verbal, although with low IQ and low functioning. His family reported that he had been doing well until 2 weeks before his admission. They stated that X enjoyed attending school, singing, and spending time with his family. He had been managed on an outpatient basis and had been doing well. X's mother reported that before this current episode X was talkative and energetic and had a bright affect. She stated that over the past few weeks she had noticed a change in his behavior, whereby he had become more withdrawn and less interactive. His mother reported possible bullying taking place at his high school because he had returned to school around the time of the onset of the episodes. His mother described episodes whereby he would lie down and become immobile and mute. She stated these episodes would last for several hours. Intermittently he would become minimally interactive and responsive but even between the episodes he did not return to his baseline.

There was a slowing in his movements and a regression in his behaviors. He was no longer able to feed himself and dress himself. He had also started urinating on the floor of the bathroom, which was not typical for him. His outpatient neurologist performed an electroencephalogram, which showed global slowing consistent with diffuse cerebral dysfunction. No epileptiform activity was noted. On admission to the hospital, routine laboratory work, including comprehensive metabolic panel, complete blood count, thyrotropin, creatine kinase, C-reactive protein, erythrocyte sedimentation rate along with MRI of brain and lumbar puncture, was performed. Cerebral spinal fluid studies for oligoclonal bands and NMDA receptor antibodies were done along with an extensive viral workup. All imaging studies and laboratory work returned normal with no significant findings. On physical examination, he was noted to have decreased strength in his upper and lower extremities bilaterally with normal flexion and extension. He had mutism and increased speech latency when he did respond. He was also noted to have blunted affect and significant psychomotor retardation.

The patient was suspected to be in pain and suffering from migraine and received lorazepam (1 mg) and a few doses of lorazepam and ketorolac tromethamine

(Toradol), which resulted in significant improvement. He was discharged after 2 days of admission, and this improvement was attributed to the pain medication. However, after being discharged, X continued to have episodes whereby he was unresponsive and minimally interactive with mutism, stupor, posturing, and staring. His family went on vacation in hopes that he would become more interactive and excited, but after a few days he began to decline further and was not able to leave the hotel room. He began refusing to eat or drink; he became incontinent, and his family had to carry him to the bathroom.

Three weeks after his previous admission, he was brought back to the emergency room with similar symptoms of muteness and severe withdrawal. A formal diagnosis of catatonia was made. He was started on lorazepam 1 mg orally twice a day, which was thought to be "too sedating" and was subsequently lowered to 0.25 mg orally 3 times a day. He began to show some improvement with lorazepam but no return to baseline. ECT was discussed with the parents as alternative and definitive treatment of catatonia. They gave consent, and he underwent an initial ECT treatment while in the hospital and showed profound improvement in his symptoms after his first treatment. He became verbal and interactive with family and visitors. He began to increase oral intake after ECT and began to be able to take care of his ADLs. He underwent a second ECT treatment during hospitalization and returned to baseline. He was discharged with scheduled maintenance ECT (M-ECT) treatments and lorazepam 0.25 mg orally 3 times a day.

At 1-year follow-up, patient X has had no relapses but has received intermittent M-ECT treatments on a flexible basis during the first 6 months whenever he started to withdraw and stops eating and drinking. During the last 6 months, he has been prescribed sertraline 100 mg per day without any further need for ECT.

Comment

This patient had a delay in formal diagnosis and appropriate treatment of catatonia, an unfortunate but not uncommon situation nowadays. There is a persistent misconception that a patient with ASD could not also have symptoms of catatonia. This misconception is probably a remnant of the longstanding but erroneous perception that catatonia is indicative of or synonymous with a schizophrenia diagnosis. Patients with ASD often have difficulty expressing symptoms, but a significant change in baseline level of functioning and behavior as seen in this case is cause for further evaluation and workup. Catatonia can be related to several psychiatric disorders, including developmental disorders, mood disorders, and substance use disorders. Catatonia is often a diagnosis of exclusion, and this may lead to a delay in treatment due to lack of awareness of the diagnosis of catatonia and how it presents. Although a medical workup was done and was found to be unremarkable, a diagnosis of catatonia was still not made, and the patient was discharged and had worsening of symptoms. Although there was some improvement with a lorazepam challenge, which is a first-line form of treatment, he required ECT treatment and M-ECT to help him return to his baseline level of functioning.

It is common to schedule ECT after the acute episode as maintenance treatment to avoid relapse and when there are incipient symptoms of catatonia. In the authors' practice, they prefer to schedule ECT on a flexible basis with open communication between the outpatient and ECT provider. Others have reported the importance of M-ECT for sustained symptom remission.[27] Ongoing ECT treatments are often imperative to prevent relapse similar as in nonautistic populations.[28,29]

Current experience supports M-ECT as an effective and safe intervention, without any sign of ensuing neuropsychological impairment, for catatonia in ASD, mirroring studies during M-ECT in general psychiatric patients showing no evidence of structural or histopathological changes,[30,31] and demonstrating similar stability of cognitive measures.[32–34]

One case series[27] presents the M-ECT courses of 3 autistic catatonic patients who received up to 286 maintenance treatments with sustained remission of catatonia and without evidence of cognitive or adaptive skill decline. In another report,[35] an autistic 21-year-old man received 220 M-ECT for catatonia over 2 years, with remarkable recovery and return to baseline psychosocial and educational functioning after severe medical compromise. His global functioning was stable throughout M-ECT, and 3 batteries of comprehensive neuropsychological functioning done yearly showed consistent stability without any evidence of cognitive decline. A further report presents an 18-year-old man with malignant catatonia in the context of congenital cerebellar dysgenesis in whom neuropsychological testing remained unchanged after 2 years following 61 M-ECT.[36]

Case Vignette 2

P is a 13-year-old male patient who was born at term after a normal pregnancy. He was diagnosed with ASD and moderate intellectual disability at the age of 3 years. He began to receive speech therapy and was enrolled in special education classes. Genetic testing was done and was found to be negative. His family history was negative. During elementary school, he was treated intermittently with stimulants for hyperactive and impulsive behaviors with good results. He also had mild tics that did not require treatment.

He participated well in school, was fluent in conversation, and able to perform his ADLs independently. In his first year of middle school, there was a sudden and sharp increase of abnormal movements, including repeated turning of the head to the left, blinking, grimacing, stuttering, repetitive movements of the fingers, and rubbing of the eyes. He started to speak less and only in a high-pitched voice. He also had waxy flexibility when examined by a neurologist who found an otherwise neurologically intact adolescent. His food and fluid intake decreased, and patient started to lose weight and sleep poorly. He had staring episodes, withdrawal, and episodes of compulsive hand washing and taking frequent showers. He became anxious and preoccupied with death and developed crying spells. His facial expression became tense and masklike. His writing skills decreased, and his grades dropped. A few weeks after onset of these symptoms, the patient disclosed that he was being bullied at school and had received a beating by other students on school grounds. His allegations were substantiated after an investigation by the school.

At the onset of these abnormal movements, 2 MRIs of the brain and an EEG were done, showing negative results. Genetic testing, including whole exome sequencing, metabolic workup, autoimmune workup (including anti-NMDAR antibodies, lupus anticoagulation therapy, antinuclear antibody panel), serum copper, and ceruloplasmin, were negative.

Over the next year, a long list of medications was prescribed by his psychiatrist targeting tics and anxiety, including several selective serotonin reuptake inhibitors (fluoxetine, sertraline), duloxetine, mirtazapine, atypical antipsychotics (risperidone, aripiprazole), fluphenazine, clonidine, guanfacine, and (low doses of) benzodiazepines (4 mg diazepam, 0.5 mg lorazepam and clonazepam) to no avail or causing side effects that necessitated discontinuation of the medication. A single dose of zolpidem (10 mg) caused agitation and increased tics.

Despite these treatments, P continued to deteriorate, needing assistance with feeding, getting dressed, brushing his teeth, and combing his hair. His speech consisted of high-pitched short sentences and remained greatly reduced. He shook his head and shattered his teeth constantly, startled in an exaggerated manner, and remained withdrawn with episodes of agitation. His neurologist diagnosed catatonia and recommended ECT, more than 1 year after onset of symptoms. ECT was not available in his state of residence due to age restrictions, causing P's family to have to travel to a neighboring state where children and adolescents are able to receive ECT treatment.

Before starting ECT, a systematic trial of lorazepam was done, starting at 1 mg twice a day with rapid escalation up to 7 mg twice a day over 10 days. Increasing the dose of lorazepam to 16 mg resulted in sedation and increased agitation. He had minimal improvement, and bilateral ECT was started on an outpatient basis, while tapering lorazepam. He improved gradually.

After 12 bilateral ECT treatments, catatonia had resolved, and the patient was functioning back at baseline. ECT was stopped and no M-ECT was required. He has not relapsed at 2-year follow-up. Maintenance treatment consists of olanzapine (25 per day) and lorazepam (6 mg per day).

Comment

This patient needed to be treated with ECT in a different state due to age-restrictive laws on ECT use in his home state despite being diagnosed there with catatonia. This anomalous and onerous legal barrier puts an undue burden on families of afflicted patients that will require remediation in the future through legal reform and overhaul by strong advocacy.[37]

Similar to the first case, a significant stressor preceded the onset of catatonic decompensation. Traumatic events and stressors are not always easily identifiable because patients with ASD may find it difficult to express this stressor due to problems with communications and conveying subjective experiences. Shah and Wing[38] also found that ongoing stressful experiences often precede the development of catatonia in autistic young adults. Life events, the loss of routine and structure, experiences of loss, conflicts with parents, caregivers, or peers, and discrepancies between the higher functioning autistic individual's capabilities and the expectations of parents can precipitate catatonia.

Observations that catatonia follows overwhelming anxiety due to trauma or perceived danger, the positive response of catatonia to anxiolytics such as benzodiazepines, and psychogenic theories of catatonia[39] are particularly applicable to people with autism due to their increased social, cognitive, and sensory vulnerabilities.[40,41] A vagal theory of catatonia in ASD has been proposed[42] as an expansion of the general polyvagal theory on the biology of social engagement and attachment first formulated by Porges in 1995[43] as a unifying framework for unifying various pathophysiological and treatment aspects of catatonia in ASD.

SUMMARY

Catatonia has been increasingly recognized in people with ASD. Assessment, diagnosis, and treatments are reviewed and illustrated in 2 new case vignettes. The use of ECT is recommended in patients who fail to respond adequately to medical treatments, including a trial of lorazepam or another benzodiazepine. The importance of M-ECT is discussed. There is an urgent need for prospective studies of catatonia in ASD and for controlled treatment trials.

ACKNOWLEDGMENTS

The authors thank the patients and their parents for letting them publish the course of their illness. The authors have omitted or changed some details to ensure anonymity.

REFERENCES

1. Billstedt E, Gilberg C, Gilberg C. Autism after adolescence: population-based 13- to 22-year follow-up study of 120 individuals with autism diagnosed in childhood. J Autism Dev Disord 2005;35:351–60.
2. Wing L, Shah A. Catatonia in autistic spectrum disorders. Br J Psychiatry 2000; 176:357–62.
3. Dhossche D, Bouman N. Catatonia in an adolescent with Prader-Willi syndrome. Ann Clin Psychiatry 1997;4:247–53.
4. Verhoeven W, Tuinier S. Prader-Willi syndrome: atypical psychoses and motor dysfunctions. Int Rev Neurobiol 2006;72:119–30.
5. Ghaziuddin N, Dhossche D, Marcotte K. Retrospective chart review of catatonia in child and adolescent psychiatric patients. Acta Psychiatr Scand 2012;125(1): 33–8.
6. Breen J, Hare DJ. The nature and prevalence of catatonic symptoms in young people with autism. J Intellect Disabil Res 2017;61(6):580–93.
7. Bell L, Oliver C, Wittkowski A, et al. Attenuated behaviour in Cornelia de Lange and fragile X syndromes. J Intellect Disabil Res 2018;62(6):486–95.
8. Wachtel LE, Griffin M, Reti I. Electroconvulsive therapy in a man with autism experiencing severe depression, catatonia, and self-Injury. J ECT 2010;96(1):70–3.
9. Wachtel LE, Jaffe R, Kellner CH. Electroconvulsive therapy for psychotropic-refractory bipolar affective disorder and severe self-injury and aggression in an 11-year-old autistic boy. Eur Child Adolesc Psychiatry 2011;20(3):147–52.
10. Volkmar F, Cohen D. Comorbid association of autism and schizophrenia. Am J Psychiatry 1991;148:1705–7.
11. Jap SN, Ghaziuddin N. Catatonia among adolescents with down syndrome: a review and 2 case reports. J ECT 2011;27(4):334–7.
12. Consoli A, Raffin M, Laurent C, et al. Medical and developmental risk factors of catatonia in children and adolescents: a prospective case-control study. Schizophr Res 2012;137(1–3):151–8.
13. American Psychiatric Association. Diagnostic and statistical manual of mental disorders, (5th Edition) (DSM-5). Washington, DC: American Psychiatric Association; 2013.
14. Kakooza-Mwesige A, Wachtel L, Dhossche D. Catatonia in autism: implications across the life span. Eur Child Adolesc Psychiatry 2008;17:327–35.
15. Dhossche D, Reti I, Wachtel L. Catatonia and autism: a historical review, with implications for ECT. J ECT 2009;25:19–22.
16. Sienaert P, Rooseleer J, De Fruyt J. Measuring catatonia: a systematic review of rating scales. J Affect Disord 2011;135(1–3):1–9.
17. Bush G, Fink M, Petrides G, et al. Catatonia: I: rating scale and standardized examination. Acta Psychiatr Scand 1996;93:129–36.
18. Bush G, Fink M, Petrides G, et al. Catatonia. II. Treatment with lorazepam and electroconvulsive therapy. Acta Psychiatr Scand 1996;93:137–43.
19. Kanner L. Autistic disturbances of affective contact. Nervous Child 1943;2: 217–50.
20. Carroll B, Kirkhart R, Ahuja N, et al. Katatonia: a new conceptual understanding of catatonia and a new rating scale. Psychiatry 2008;5:42–50.
21. Oliver C, Licence L, Richards C. Self-injurious behaviour in people with intellectual disability and autism spectrum disorder. Curr Opin Psychiatry 2017;30(2): 97–101.

22. Matson JL, Lovullo SV. A review of behavioral treatments for self-injurious behaviors of persons with autism spectrum disorders. Behav Modif 2008;32(1): 61–76.

23. Wing L, Shah A. A systematic examination of catatonic-like clinical pictures in autism spectrum disorders. Int Rev Neurobiol 2006;72:21–39.

24. Wachtel LE, Dhossche DM. Self-injury in autism as an alternate sign of catatonia: implications for electroconvulsive therapy. Med Hypotheses 2010;75(1):111–4.

25. Wachtel L, Dhossche D. ECT for self-injurious behavior. In: Ghaziuddin M, Walter G, editors. Electroconvulsive therapy in children and adolescents. New York: Oxord University Press; 2013. p. 247–80.

26. DeJong H, Bunton P, Hare DJ. A systematic review of interventions used to treat catatonic symptoms in people with autistic spectrum disorders. J Autism Dev Disord 2014;44(9):2127–36.

27. Wachtel LE, Hermida A, Dhossche DM. Maintenance electroconvulsive therapy in autistic catatonia: a case series review. Prog Neuropsychopharmacol Biol Psychiatry 2010;34(4):581–7.

28. Kellner C, Knapp R, Petrides G, et al. Continuation electroconvulsive therapy vs pharmacotherapy for relapse prevention in major depression: a multisite study from the Consortium for Research in Electroconvulsive Therapy (CORE). Arch Gen Psychiatry 2006;63:1337–44.

29. Petrides G, Dhossche D, Fink M, et al. Continuation ECT: relapse prevention in affective disorders. Convuls Ther 1994;10:189–94.

30. Lippman S, Manshadi M, Wehry M, et al. 1,250 electroconvulsive treatments without evidence of brain injury. Br J Psychiatry 1985;147:203–4.

31. Scalia J, Lisanby SH, Dwork AJ, et al. Neuropathologic examination after 91 ECT treatments in a 92-year-old woman with late-onset depression. J ECT 2007;23(2): 96–8.

32. Devanand DP, Verma AK, Tirumalasetti F, et al. Absence of cognitive impairment after more than 100 lifetime ECT treatments. Am J Psychiatry 1991;148(7): 929–32.

33. Wijkstra J, Nolen WA. Successful maintenance electroconvulsive therapy for more than seven years. J ECT 2005;21(3):171–3.

34. Zisselman M, Rosenquist P, Curlik S. Long-term weekly continuation electroconvulsive therapy: a case-series. J ECT 2007;23:274–7.

35. Wachtel LE, Reti IM, Dhossche DM, et al. Stability of neuropsychological testing during two years of maintenance electroconvulsive therapy in an autistic man. Prog Neuropsychopharmacol Biol Psychiatry 2011;35(1):301–2.

36. Wachtel D, Dhossche D, Reti IM, et al. Stability of neuropsychological testing during maintenance electroconvulsive therapy. Pediatr Neurol 2012;47(3): 219–21.

37. Wachtel LE, Dhossche DM. Challenges of electroconvulsive therapy for catatonia in youth with intellectual disabilities: another tomato effect? J ECT 2012;28(3): 151–3.

38. Shah A, Wing L. Psychological approaches to chronic catatonia-like deterioration in autism spectrum disorders. Int Rev Neurobiol 2006;72:245–64.

39. Moskowitz AK. "Scared stiff": catatonia as an evolutionary-based fear response. Psychol Rev 2004;111(4):984–1002.

40. Dhossche DM, Ross CA, Stoppelbein L. The role of deprivation, abuse, and trauma in pediatric catatonia without a clear medical cause. Acta Psychiatr Scand 2012;125(1):25–32.

41. Dhossche D. Catatonia: the ultimate yet treatable motor reaction to fear in autism. Autism 2011;1:103. https://doi.org/10.4172/2165-7890.1000103.
42. Dhossche D. Autonomic dysfunction in catatonia in autism: implications of a vagal theory. Autism 2012;2:e114. https://doi.org/10.4172/2165-7890.1000e114.
43. Porges SW. Social engagement and attachment: a phylogenetic perspective. Ann N Y Acad Sci 2003;1008:31–47.

Electroconvulsive Therapy for Catatonia in Children and Adolescents

Dirk M. Dhossche, MD, PhD[a],*, Nisha Withane, MD[b]

KEYWORDS

- Catatonia • Children • Adolescents • Pediatric • Electroconvulsive treatment (ECT)
- Benzodiazepines

KEY POINTS

- In its malignant form, catatonia features autonomic dysfunction including fever, and becomes an acute, potentially life-threatening disorder; however, it is a treatable condition that warrants prompt diagnosis and treatment with benzodiazepines as first-line treatment and electroconvulsive treatment as definitive treatment.
- Catatonia develops in children and adolescents with concurrent medical conditions, including lupus and anti–N-methyl-D-aspartic acid receptor encephalitis, psychotic and affective disorders, toxic states, autism spectrum disorders, developmental disorders, tic disorders, posttraumatic conditions, and miscellaneous syndromes such as Kleine-Levin syndrome and pervasive refusal syndrome.
- To reduce morbidity and mortality in patients with catatonia and to increase further research, the Diagnostic and Statistical Manual of Mental Disorders, 5th edition, changed the classification of catatonia.
- Clinical experience and case-reports support benzodiazepines and electroconvulsive therapy (ECT), including maintenance ECT, as safe and effective treatments for pediatric catatonia that do not carry the risk for precipitating neuroleptic malignant syndrome.
- The mechanism of catatonia is unknown, yet the vagal theory may lead to better understanding and new treatments.

INTRODUCTION

Catatonia is a severe and potentially life-threatening acute illness, especially in its malignant form when it is accompanied by autonomic dysfunction and high fevers; however, it is treatable when recognized and treated promptly.[1] It occurs in children and adolescents, as in adults, in a variety of forms, including medical and autoimmune

Disclosure Statement: The authors have no conflicts of interest.
[a] Department of Psychiatry, University of Mississippi Medical Center, 2500 North State Street, Jackson, MS 39216, USA; [b] Department of Psychiatry, Institute of Living/Hartford Hospital, 200 Retreat Avenue, Hartford, CT 06114, USA
* Corresponding author.
E-mail address: dirkdhossche@gmail.com

Child Adolesc Psychiatric Clin N Am 28 (2019) 111–120
https://doi.org/10.1016/j.chc.2018.07.007
1056-4993/19/© 2018 Elsevier Inc. All rights reserved.

diseases, such as lupus[2-4] or anti–N-methyl-D-aspartic acid (anti-NMDA) receptor encephalitis[5-7]; psychotic and affective disorders; toxic states, such as neuroleptic malignant syndrome (NMS); autism spectrum disorders (ASDs); developmental disorders; tic disorders; posttraumatic conditions; and miscellaneous syndromes, such as Kleine-Levin syndrome and pervasive refusal syndrome (PRS).[8,9]

Prevalence studies of pediatric catatonia show a very wide range of estimates that are likely due to differences in study samples and methods of assessment. Two studies find catatonia in 12% to 17% of adolescents and young adults with ASD.[10,11] The highest rate is noted in a sample of adolescents referred for electroconvulsive therapy (ECT) in which almost half (45%) had catatonia.[12] In another study,[13] catatonia was found in 18% of adolescents who were admitted to a psychiatric hospital and who had known risk factors for catatonia, such as a diagnosis of pervasive developmental disorder, atypical psychosis, intermittent explosive disorder, mental retardation, catatonia, or NMS. Their treatment providers had diagnosed only 2 subjects with catatonia. These findings mirror studies in adult general psychiatric subjects, which report low rates of catatonia between 1% and 24%.[1] Overall, these findings support the view that catatonia may be more common in children, adolescents, and adults than previously thought.

There are no controlled studies on the use of benzodiazepines or ECT in children and adolescents. Clinical experience and case-reports support benzodiazepines and ECT, including maintenance ECT, as safe and effective treatments for pediatric catatonia that do not carry the risk for precipitating NMS.[8,9] In general psychiatric adult patients, benzodiazepines are effective in more than half of cases, up to 80%, and the remaining patients uniformly respond to ECT.

DIAGNOSTIC CLASSIFICATION UPDATE BOOSTS THE RECOGNITION OF PEDIATRIC CATATONIA

The *Diagnostic and Statistical Manual of Mental Disorders*, 5th edition, (DSM-5), published a few years ago,[14] includes changes in the classification of catatonia that aim to reduce morbidity and mortality in patients with catatonia and to increase further research. The DSM-5 catatonia classification features 3 main categories: catatonia associated with another mental disorder (293.89), catatonic disorder due to another medical condition (293.89), and unspecified catatonia (781.99 and 293.89). The uncoupling of catatonia and schizophrenia is important for increasing recognition of catatonia as a separate condition that may require separate treatment apart from the wide range of comorbid conditions, including in children and adolescents.

All 3 diagnoses use the same definition of catatonia and require that 3 out of 12 symptoms are present.[14] Symptoms include (1) catalepsy (passive induction of a posture held against gravity), (2) waxy flexibility (during reposturing patients offers initial resistance before allowing himself or herself to be repositioned, similar to that of bending a warm candle), (3) stupor (extreme hypoactivity, immobility, minimally responsive to stimuli), (4) agitation (extreme hyperactivity, constant motor unrest that appears nonpurposeful), (5) mutism (verbally unresponsive or minimally responsive), (6) negativism (apparently motiveless resistance to instructions or to attempts to move or examine the patient, or contrary behavior in which the patient does the opposite of the instruction), (7) posturing (maintains postures, including mundane; eg, sitting or standing for hours without reacting), (8) mannerisms (odd, purposeful movements, such as hopping or walking tiptoe, saluting passers-by, exaggerated caricatures of mundane movements), (9) stereotypies (repetitive, not goal-directed, motor activity; eg, finger-play or repeatedly touching, patting, or rubbing self), (10) grimacing (maintenance of odd facial expressions), (11) echolalia (mimicking of examiner's speech), or (12) echopraxia (mimicking of examiner's movements).

NMS is recognized in the DSM-5 as the drug-induced form of malignant catatonia. The DSM-5 text reads[14]: "Catatonia can be a side-effect of medication. Because of the seriousness of the complications, particular attention should be paid to the possibility that catatonia is attributable to NMS. Individuals with schizophrenia or a mood disorder may present with malignant catatonia indistinguishable from NMS. Some investigators consider NMS to be a drug-induced form of malignant catatonia."

The new DSM-5 category, unspecified catatonia, is recommended for patients for whom the general medical condition contributing to catatonia may not be identified initially but whose level of impairment warrants specific treatment of catatonia (eg, patients who develop catatonia in the context of autoimmune and paraneoplastic disorders, such as anti-NMDA receptor encephalitis); for pediatric patients with catatonia; and for patients with catatonia with ASD, other neurodevelopmental disorders, and other conditions, such as tic disorders and Tourette syndrome, Kleine-Levin syndrome, posttraumatic reactions, and PRS.

ASSESSMENT AND TREATMENT

Catatonia should be suspected early on when psychomotor retardation, agitation, or other motor symptoms are prominent. Mutism, stereotypic speech, echolalia, stereotypic or repetitive behaviors, posturing, grimacing, rigidity, mannerisms, and purposeless agitation are present in various combinations. Several catatonic symptoms overlap with autistic symptoms, yet autistic patients qualify for a diagnosis of catatonia when there is a sharp increase of these symptoms with marked departure from baseline function.[11,15] In some autistic patients, catatonia crystalizes into frenzied compulsive self-injurious behavior.[16,17]

A medical workup is useful to rule out other concomitant conditions and includes blood work with basic hematologic and basic measures, comprehensive drug testing, brain imaging, autoimmune antibodies (lupus serology, PANDAS serology, anti-NMDA receptor antibodies), and other tests guided by clinical examinations.

Most children and adolescents with catatonia do not have any underlying definable medical condition. For example, in a sample of 58 children and adolescents with catatonia,[18] 13 (22%) subjects had medical conditions and 18 (31%) had a history of developmental disorder, such as ASD, intellectual disability, or neurodevelopmental malformation. Medical conditions ($n = 13$) associated with catatonia included autoimmune encephalitis (systemic lupus erythematous [$N = 3$] and anti-NMDA receptor encephalitis [$n = 1$]), seizures ($n = 1$), cyclosporine encephalitis ($n = 1$), posthypoglycemic coma encephalitis ($n = 1$), and genetic or metabolic conditions (chorea [$n = 2$] 5-hydroxytryptamine [5-HT] cerebrospinal fluid deficit [$n = 1$], storage disease [$n = 1$], fatal familial insomnia [$n = 1$], and PRODH (proline dehydrogenase) mutations [$n = 1$]). Only 2 subjects with a history of developmental disorder had an identifiable underlying medical or psychiatric condition.

Antipsychotics should be avoided owing to the risk of worsening catatonia or precipitating NMS. A rating scale for estimating severity can assist in diagnosis.

A positive lorazepam test validates catatonia. If catatonia improves considerably after a 1 or 2 mg test dose of lorazepam taken per oral (po); intramuscularly (IM); or, ideally, intravenously (IV), then lorazepam should be continued and titrated rapidly for optimal response and maintenance of improvement, often to dosages between 10 and 30 mg per day. Surprisingly, these higher doses do not exert expected sedating effects in many catatonic patients, unlike in patients without catatonia, probably reflecting particular abnormalities of gamma-aminobutyric acid (GABA) function or the GABA-benzodiazepine receptor. An alternative to lorazepam is zolpidem, 5 to 10 mg, which is only available in po form.

If there is no response, bilateral ECT should be initiated. The use of bilateral (bitem-poral or bifrontal) electrode placement is recommended as the most effective method compared with other methods of electrode placement. The number and frequency of treatments is often higher in the treatment of catatonia than in affective disorders. Sometimes daily en bloc treatments are needed for 3 to 5 consecutive days in severe cases with malignant catatonia. Sometimes improvement occurs quickly but in some patients 10 to 20 treatments are needed. The presence of autonomic instability in catatonia indicates malignant catatonia, an urgent call for ECT.[19]

Acute ECT may be followed by continuation ECT to avoid relapses. After a few more treatments, some patients do not require any further treatment. Others require main-tenance ECT to avoid relapses. Current experience supports maintenance ECT as an effective and safe intervention for pediatric catatonia or catatonia in ASD,[20–22] without any signs of ensuing neuropsychological impairment.

Concomitant psychiatric or medical conditions may require separate treatment after treatment of catatonia is initiated and major catatonic impairment is dissipating.

MECHANISMS OF CATATONIA AND NEW VAGAL THEORY

De Jong and Barruk[23] were pioneers experimental catatonia. In 1928, they induced catatonia in animals by bulbocapnine, an alkaloid found in the plant family Fumaria-ceae, which acts as an acetylcholinesterase inhibitor by increasing cholinergic tone and inhibiting biosynthesis of dopamine via inhibition of the enzyme tyrosine hydrox-ylase. The occurrence of catatonia in such a bewildering range of conditions and its unique response to benzodiazepines and ECT support the view that catatonia has unique biological correlates separate from other conditions. A unifying pathogenesis of catatonia remains elusive although there are several models of catatonia.[24] Current theories suggest motor circuitry, epilepsy, neurotransmitters, genetics, endocri-nology, immunology, and traumatic fear.

The fear model of catatonia is based on the animal reflex of tonic immobility[25] and is supported by observations that catatonia can develop after severe traumatic events or perceived danger, also in children and adolescents,[26] by the positive response of catatonia to anxiolytics such as benzodiazepines or barbiturates, and by psychogenic theories of catatonia.[27] A vagal theory of catatonia has been proposed[28,29] as an expansion of the general polyvagal theory on the biology of social engagement and attachment, detachment, and freezing response, in the fight-flight-freeze survival cascade, first formulated by Porges[30] in 1995. The vagal theory of catatonia unifies some various aspects of catatonia and stimulates further studies on autonomic dysfunction and the use of anticholinergic agents and, at least theoretically, vagal nerve stimulation.[29] Acetylcholine is the principal neurotransmitter released at target organs by the vagal nerve and there are a few indications in the literature that the anti-cholinergic medications biperiden and benztropine may acutely relieve catatonia as described in case reports.[31,32] Further studies on anticholinergic agents and catatonia are warranted in view of the vagal theory. It is currently unknown if vagal nerve stim-ulatory techniques as currently used in refractory seizure disorders are effective in catatonia.

Case Vignette 1

J is an 11-year-old girl with a history of attention-deficit hyperactivity disorder and anxiety disorder who presented to the emergency room with altered mental status. Her parents reported that she had become more confused, almost stopped speaking, and had spells of crying and screaming. She had become more irritable, more anxious, sleepless, and minimally interactive and cooperative, which was not typical for her. The patient had begun neglecting her hygiene, had difficulty feeding herself, and had an overall regression. She was followed by an outpatient psychiatrist who had been prescribing lorazepam 0.5 mg po every bedtime (qhs), melatonin 6 mg po qhs, and aripiprazole 15 mg po daily before her admission.

She was admitted to the pediatric hospital and both neurology and psychiatry were consulted. She was started on IV fluids because of her poor oral intake and an infectious workup was ordered. Laboratory tests were conducted for cytomegalovirus, Epstein-Barr virus, human immunodeficiency virus, Bartonella, Mycoplasma, and Lyme disease. Paraneoplastic workup, including anti-NMDA receptor antibodies, MRI, and magnetic resonance angiography studies were all negative. Corticosteroids and IV immunoglobulin therapy (IVIG) were started by neurology for a putative diagnosis of autoimmune encephalitis (although no positive antibodies were found). She showed no improvement after 1 week of treatment. Nuedexta (dextromethorphan hydrobromide and quinidine sulfate) was started for possible pseudobulbar affect with no improvement. Lorazepam was titrated up to 3 mg every 6 hours with minimal improvement, although she tolerated this high dose of lorazepam well without any signs of sedation or side effects.

J continued to have poor oral intake and symptoms of mutism, posturing, psychomotor retardation, stupor, and echolalia, qualifying for a diagnosis of catatonia. Psychiatry recommended a trial of ECT for symptoms of catatonia. J's parents consented to ECT treatment and she received ECT bitemporal ECT treatments 3 times per week. She began to show rapid and significant improvement with speech, eating, movement, ambulation, and mood starting after the first ECT. Catatonia resolved after 6 treatments over 2 weeks and she was discharged from the hospital with plans for continuation ECT.

During the 2-year follow-up after the acute treatment course, J has had no relapses but has continued on a flexible schedule of maintenance ECT, ranging 2 to 4 weeks between sessions. The parents are reluctant to stop ECT maintenance all together owing to fears and risks of relapse with the need for acute hospitalization. J experiences no physical or cognitive side effects of ECT, except the occasional headache during the day of ECT. Her social and educational development is progressing well. No medical issues have arisen.

Comment

This young adolescent met criteria for catatonia, that is, psychomotor slowing, inability to walk, decreased food and fluid intake, episodes of agitation and screaming (seemingly purposeless). Other symptoms, such as echolalia, echopraxia, and waxy flexibility were not present. ECT proved to be the definitive treatment with an astoundingly fast response, whereas immune treatments (corticosteroids and IVIG) and high-dose benzodiazepine treatment (up to 12 mg per day) failed to improve her condition.

ECT was an effective and safe maintenance treatment in this case. However, there are no published guidelines on how often and how long ECT can or should continue. The patient and her parents were motivated to continue with ECT; however, at some time in the future, as the patient remains without signs of relapse, ECT should be tapered and stopped.

Further follow-up should be informative on the diagnosis in this patient. It is unclear at this time if her catatonic decompensation 2 years earlier will prove to be a harbinger of a mood disorder or another major psychiatric syndrome or will remain an isolated event. Previous studies have shown that catatonia is common in the manic phase of bipolar illness.[33]

Another diagnostic consideration in this case concerns the presence of insomnia, emotional lability, dysphoria, anxiety, episodes of frenzied crying, and perplexed mood, pointing to the mood abnormalities in a patient with catatonia. Other investigators have reported the combination of mood lability, perplexity, and signs of confusion and delirium in patients with catatonia, and have coined the presentation variously as manic delirium, delirious mania, catatonic mania, and excited catatonia, all with excellent response to ECT.[34]

CASE VIGNETTE 2

K is a 15-year-old boy who presented to the hospital for altered mental status. His family reported that he had smoked what he called a cigarette in the afternoon, then fell backwards, began foaming at the mouth, and had an undetectable pulse. A friend who was passing by started chest compressions and K became responsive. He was taken to the local emergency room for evaluation and discharged after a few hours. K continued to have altered mental status and was minimally interactive and responsive and he was taken to a larger general hospital for further evaluation. In the emergency room, he was only responsive to pain or noxious stimuli. His speech was incoherent and nonsensical and his family reported he was not functioning at his baseline. Imaging studies were done, including a computed tomography (CT) head, an electroencephalogram (EEG), and an echocardiogram, as well as basic laboratory tests. Neurology was consulted but CT head imaging and EEG were normal studies and no further neurologic workup was required. He was admitted for altered mental status and suspected episodes of catatonia in which the patient showed symptoms of selective mutism, posturing, immobility, and staring. His sister reported that during his first night in the hospital, he stared at the television all night with decreased blinking and limited visual scanning. His laboratory work showed a urine drug screen positive for cannabinoids, an elevated creatine kinase of 430, and an elevated creatinine of 0.88. Other laboratory work was grossly unremarkable. He was also noted to have decreased oral intake.

During the course of hospitalization, K admitted that he had used so-called spice and was also using marijuana regularly. Psychiatry was consulted for suspected catatonia. The psychiatric consultant stated that he had endorsed symptoms of depression but documented that his psychiatric examination showed that he was minimally interactive with little movement. He was unable to feed himself and had increased latency with speech when responding. He had a restricted affect and was not very interactive. The psychiatrist believed the symptoms were due to a substance-induced delirium and did not think further intervention was required, apart from haloperidol as needed for agitation. A trial of lorazepam was not done despite significant symptoms for suspected catatonia and the patient was discharged home after 4 days.

K did not return to baseline according to his family. After 2 weeks, his symptoms worsened and he began to display even more prominently catatonic features of mutism, immobility, and severe psychomotor retardation. His family reported that he had been lying in his bed for 4 days with minimal interaction or movement. He was admitted for psychosis and started on olanzapine (up to 10 mg per day) and lorazepam 0.5 mg daily. He was also started on subcutaneous enoxaparin sodium (Lovenox) 40 mg daily for deep vein thrombosis (DVT) prophylaxis. He showed minimal improvement after 1 month, continued to have episodes of catatonia, and was finally transferred to a psychiatric hospital for further evaluation and treatment.

On arrival, K was noted to have mutism, facial grimacing, immobility, and staring, and catatonia was recognized and diagnosed as such. Olanzapine was discontinued. Subcutaneous enoxaparin sodium was continued. He was given a 2 mg IM lorazepam challenge and showed moderate improvement but symptoms returned after a few hours. Lorazepam was then started and scheduled every 6 hours. He was placed on fall precautions and seizure precautions. He was also ordered a safety belt with his wheelchair and a helmet to prevent any head injuries due to him being unable to walk unassisted. He required the staff's assistance to help him with all of his activities of daily living.

Lorazepam was titrated up to 18 mg per day (6 mg po 3 times a day [tid]) and K only showed mild to moderate improvement but no sedation or any other side effects. K remained mute and did not respond to questions. He displayed waxy flexibility and posturing. He also began to have symptoms of echolalia and used high-pitched mimicking of speech. Lorazepam was stopped and replaced with zolpidem 15 mg po tid with some improvement as he became more interactive and was seen walking with assistance of the staff, laughing, and waving at peers. He was still unable to follow directions from the staff or follow commands appropriately. Adding methylphenidate (up to 15 mg tid) during a 5 day period did not have any effect.

Although improvement of the most severe symptoms of catatonia was evident with treatment with sedative treatment (lorazepam and zolpidem) because K started to eat and drink more (mostly with assistance) and was no longer bedridden, he did not return to baseline 2 weeks into this admission and about 2.5 months into his illness. ECT was discussed with the mother as the best option for expedient resolution of catatonia and she provided informed consent.

Bitemporal ECT was started and well-tolerated. After the first ECT treatment, K continued to be mute but began to answer questions by writing down his answers. He wrote that he did not remember how long he had been in the hospital. He continued 2 more ECT treatments and became fully interactive, speaking with peers and staff. He began talking about his favorite sport and the position he played. He was able to eat on his own without any assistance from staff. He also began to ambulate on his own. K began to participate in school and group activities and received a total of 6 ECT treatments before complete resolution of catatonia. Two weeks after the start of ECT, he was discharged home to the delight of his family. The only medication prescribed was clonazepam 4 mg po qhs. No maintenance ECT was scheduled. At 1-year follow-up, there have been no relapses.

Comment

ECT was the definitive treatment in this case, with catatonia probably induced by synthetic cannabinoids (spice). Other investigators have reported the association between this type of toxic psychosis and catatonia and its response to ECT.[35–37] The authors found no studies in the literature that have systematically assessed the presence of catatonia, malignant catatonia, or NMS, in cases suspected with spice-induced psychosis.

Recommended treatments for catatonia were not started for several months, despite the documented presence of catatonia in the medical records, until his third admission about 2 months into his illness. Prior psychiatric evaluations mentioned delirium, psychosis, mood disorder, selective mutism, adjustment disorder, and substance-induced psychosis but not catatonia. He was not given a lorazepam challenge and he continued to be treated with antipsychotic medications and a subtherapeutic dose of lorazepam before his third admission in which full-blown catatonia was formally diagnosed and treated accordingly with rapid resolution.

Catatonia can lead to serious and life-threatening complications, including infections and DVT due to immobility, dehydration, and muscle breakdown due to decreased oral intake. Catatonia in this case was related to substance use, most likely adulterated or synthetic marijuana, but did not resolve and persisted for several weeks due to lack of appropriate recognition and treatment.

DISCUSSION

Prediction is very difficult, especially if it's about the future.
    —Niels Bohr (1885–1962, Danish 1922 Nobel laureate in Physics)

Catatonic presentations in children and adolescents warrant attention given the rich history of catatonia in psychiatry, yet current state of underrecognition across all psychiatry and medicine[38]; its occurrence in a wide age range; its easily recognizable signature of the combination of motor and autonomic symptoms; its considerable morbidity and mortality; and, most importantly, its prompt and profound response to sedative treatment (benzodiazepines and zolpidem) and ECT. Witnessing the quick resolution of catatonia by benzodiazepines and ECT in patients, both pediatric and adult, leaves an indelible mark on clinicians and health workers, and brings relief to the family, as shown in the 2 new case-vignettes presented.

The DSM-5 promotes the significance of catatonia, yet fails to give it hierarchical diagnostic and treatment priority compared with chronic and amorphous medical and psychiatric conditions for which optimal treatment is unclear. Psychiatrists learn about catatonia, yet do not often encounter cases if they practice outside acute settings. Nonpsychiatric specialists come across cases of catatonia in medical settings but do not recognize the syndrome and instead label it as autoimmune (anti-NMDA) receptor encephalitis, delirium, or regression; and are less versed in the use of benzodiazepine challenges or ECT. The prompt applications of a trial of benzodiazepines and ECT are currently problematic. Conducting a trial of benzodiazepines, with titration to levels often higher than recommended for anxiety, requires a focused and deliberate effort. Referral to ECT is compromised at times for various reasons, including by local, state (in the United States), or national (in some countries) laws with age-restrictions on ECT use.

There are no systematic studies on catatonia in children and adolescents, yet assessment and treatment rests on solid clinical and empirical bases. Dedicated research on catatonia is warranted because current evidence supports that pediatric catatonia is a treatable condition when recognized early and treated accordingly.

ACKNOWLEDGMENTS

The authors thank the patients and their parents for allowing us to publish this article about the course of their illnesses. We have omitted or changed some details to ensure anonymity.

REFERENCES

1. Fink M. Rediscovering catatonia: the biography of a treatable syndrome. Acta Psychiatr Scand Suppl 2013;(441):1–47.
2. Ali A, Taj A, Uz-Zehra M. Lupus catatonia in a young girl who presented with fever and altered sensorium. Pak J Med Sci 2014;30(2):446–8.
3. Leon T, Aguirre A, Pesce C, et al. Electroconvulsive therapy for catatonia in juvenile neuropsychiatric lupus. Lupus 2014;23(10):1066–8.
4. Mon T, L'Ecuyer S, Farber NB, et al. The use of electroconvulsive therapy in a patient with juvenile systemic lupus erythematosus and catatonia. Lupus 2012; 21(14):1575–81.
5. Dhossche D, Fink M, Shorter E, et al. Anti-NMDA receptor encephalitis versus pediatric catatonia. Am J Psychiatry 2011;168(7):749–50.
6. Wilson JE, Shuster J, Fuchs C. Anti-NMDA receptor encephalitis in a 14-year-old female presenting as malignant catatonia: medical and psychiatric approach to treatment. Psychosomatics 2013;54(6):585–9.
7. Kanbayashi T, Tsutsui K, Tanaka K, et al. Anti-NMDA encephalitis in psychiatry; malignant catatonia, atypical psychosis and ECT. Rinsho Shinkeigaku 2014; 54(12):1103–6 [in Japanese].
8. Dhossche D, Wilson C, Wachtel L. Catatonia in childhood and adolescence: implications for the DSM-5. Prim Psychiatry 2010;17:35–9.
9. Dhossche DM, Wachtel LE. Catatonia is hidden in plain sight among different pediatric disorders: a review article. Pediatr Neurol 2010;43(5):307–15.

10. Billstedt E, Gilberg C, Gilberg C. Autism after adolescence: population-based 13-to 22-year follow-up study of 120 individuals with autism diagnosed in childhood. J Autism Dev Disord 2005;35:351–60.
11. Wing L, Shah A. Catatonia in autistic spectrum disorders. Br J Psychiatry 2000;176:357–62.
12. Moise FN, Petrides G. Case study: electroconvulsive therapy in adolescents. J Am Acad Child Adolesc Psychiatry 1996;35(3):312–8.
13. Ghaziuddin N, Dhossche D, Marcotte K. Retrospective chart review of catatonia in child and adolescent psychiatric patients. Acta Psychiatr Scand 2012;125(1):33–8.
14. American Psychiatric Association. Diagnostic and statistical manual of mental disorders, (5th edition) (DSM-5). Washington, DC: American Psychiatric Association; 2013.
15. Dhossche DM. Decalogue of catatonia in autism spectrum disorders. Front Psychiatry 2014;5:157.
16. Wachtel LE, Contrucci-Kuhn SA, Griffin M, et al. ECT for self-injury in an autistic boy. Eur Child Adolesc Psychiatry 2009;18(7):458–63.
17. Wachtel LE, Dhossche DM. Self-injury in autism as an alternate sign of catatonia: implications for electroconvulsive therapy. Med Hypotheses 2010;75(1):111–4.
18. Consoli A, Raffin M, Laurent C, et al. Medical and developmental risk factors of catatonia in children and adolescents: a prospective case-control study. Schizophr Res 2012;137(1–3):151–8.
19. Wachtel L, Commins E, Park M, et al. Neuroleptic malignant syndrome and delirious mania as malignant catatonia in autism: prompt relief with electroconvulsive therapy. Acta Psychiatr Scand 2015;132(4):319–20.
20. Wachtel LE, Hermida A, Dhossche DM. Maintenance electroconvulsive therapy in autistic catatonia: a case series review. Prog Neuropsychopharmacol Biol Psychiatry 2010;34(4):581–7.
21. Consoli A, Cohen J, Bodeau N, et al. Electroconvulsive therapy in adolescents with intellectual disability and severe self-injurious behavior and aggression: a retrospective study. Eur Child Adolesc Psychiatry 2013;22(1):55–62.
22. Wachtel D, Dhossche D, Reti IM, et al. Stability of neuropsychological testing during maintenance electroconvulsive therapy. Pediatr Neurol 2012;47(3):219–21.
23. De Jong HH, Barruk H. A clinical and experimental study of the catatonic syndrome (Étude comparative expérimentale et clinique des manifestations du syndrome catatonique). Rev Neurol 1929;1:21–34.
24. Dhossche DM, Stoppelbein L, Rout UK. Etiopathogenesis of catatonia: generalizations and working hypotheses. J ECT 2010;26(4):253–8.
25. Gallup G, Maser J. Tonic immobility: evolutionary underpinnings of human catalepsy and catatonia. In: Maser J, Seligman M, editors. Psychopathology: experimental models. San Francisco (CA): Freeman; 1977. p. 334–57.
26. Dhossche DM, Ross CA, Stoppelbein L. The role of deprivation, abuse, and trauma in pediatric catatonia without a clear medical cause. Acta Psychiatr Scand 2012;125(1):25–32.
27. Moskowitz AK. "Scared stiff": catatonia as an evolutionary-based fear response. Psychol Rev 2004;111(4):984–1002.
28. Dhossche D. Autonomic dysfunction in catatonia in autism: implications of a vagal theory. Autism Open Access 2012;2(4). https://doi.org/10.4172/2165-7890.1000e114.
29. Dhossche DM. Vagal intimations for catatonia and electroconvulsive therapy. J ECT 2014;30(2):111–5.

30. Porges SW. Social engagement and attachment: a phylogenetic perspective. Ann N Y Acad Sci 2003;1008:31–47.

31. Franz M, Gallhofer B, Kanzow WT. Treatment of catatonia with intravenous biperidene. Br J Psychiatry 1994;164(6):847–8.

32. Albucher RC, DeQuardo J, Tandon R. Treatment of catatonia with an anticholinergic agent. Biol Psychiatry 1991;29(5):513–4.

33. Taylor MA, Abrams R. Catatonia. Prevalence and importance in the manic phase of manic-depressive illness. Arch Gen Psychiatry 1977;34(10):1223–5.

34. Fink M. Delirious mania. Bipolar Disord 1999;1(1):54–60.

35. Haro G, Ripoll C, Ibanez M, et al. Could spice drugs induce psychosis with abnormal movements similar to catatonia? Psychiatry 2014;77(2):206–8.

36. Leibu E, Garakani A, McGonigle DP, et al. Electroconvulsive therapy (ECT) for catatonia in a patient with schizophrenia and synthetic cannabinoid abuse: a case report. J ECT 2013;29(4):e61–2.

37. Smith DL, Roberts C. Synthetic marijuana use and development of catatonia in a 17-year-old male. Minn Med 2014;97(5):38.

38. Llesuy JR, Medina M, Jacobson KC, et al. Catatonia under-diagnosis in the general hospital. J Neuropsychiatry Clin Neurosci 2018;30(2):145–51.

Electroconvulsive Therapy as a Safe, Effective Treatment for Catatonia in an Adolescent with a Nasogastric Tube: A Case Report

Paul A. Fuchs, MD, MPH*, Todd E. Peters, MD,
Margaret M. Benningfield, MD

KEYWORDS

• ECT • Adolescent • Nasogastric tube • Feeding tube • Neuromodulation

KEY POINTS

- Electroconvulsive therapy is a safe, effective treatment for many psychiatric disorders, is especially effective for the treatment of catatonia, and has no absolute contraindications.
- Stigma surrounding electroconvulsive therapy can be a significant barrier to appropriate care for patients and likely influences institutional policies.
- Having a feeding tube should not be treated as an absolute contraindication to electroconvulsive therapy.

INTRODUCTION

There are many obstacles to appropriate psychiatric care. In American society, stigma surrounds even the least invasive treatments, such as psychotherapy. Encouraging patients to take medications for their mental illness, can be difficult. Often, when a patient requires a more invasive treatment, such as electroconvulsive therapy (ECT), the stigma is too much to overcome.

Much of the stigma surrounding ECT stems from misinformation and historical methodology. When ECT was first developed for the treatment of psychiatric illnesses in the 1930s, it was administered bilaterally using a sinusoidal waveform, which has

Disclosure Statement: Dr T. Peters serves as the Consulting Editor for *Child and Adolescent Psychiatric Clinics of North America*. Dr P.A. Fuchs and Dr M.M. Benningfield have no disclosures to report.
Department of Psychiatry and Behavioral Sciences, Vanderbilt University Medical Center, 1601 23rd Avenue South, Nashville, TN 37212, USA
* Corresponding author.
E-mail address: paul.a.fuchs@vumc.org

Child Adolesc Psychiatric Clin N Am 28 (2019) 121–125
https://doi.org/10.1016/j.chc.2018.08.002
1056-4993/19/© 2018 Elsevier Inc. All rights reserved.

Abbreviation	
ECT	Electroconvulsive therapy

greater risk for side effects. In addition, the early use of ECT was not done with anesthesia, muscle relaxants, or supplemental oxygen, further increasing the risk of physical harm to the patient (eg, fractures). At times, patients were administered the treatment without adhering to modern standards of informed consent, because the standards were not developed by the American Psychiatric Association until 1978.[1,2] Although current methodology and ethical standards differs significantly from early practice, the stigma remains.

Briefly, ECT involves applying an electric current to the patient's brain to induce a controlled seizure under anesthesia and has been shown to be an effective treatment for depression, bipolar affective disorder, schizophrenia, schizoaffective disorder, neuroleptic malignant syndrome, and catatonia.[3]

Catatonia comprises a constellation of symptoms marked by abnormal activity that often present with increased or decreased motor movements, muscle tone, and abnormal posturing, among other symptoms.[4] Catatonia is thought to be a complication of an underlying psychiatric or physical illness, and can be associated with psychosis, depression, or autoimmune diseases such as systemic lupus erythematosus, among other illnesses.[4–6] Although some catatonic patients can be medically managed with benzodiazepines, ECT remains one of the most effective treatments for catatonia and has no absolute contraindications.[3,4]

Although patients and families of patients who have received ECT tend to have a positive perception of the treatment,[7,8] ECT remains stigmatized and it can be difficult to find a provider willing and certified to perform ECT. In many areas of the country, there are limited numbers of ECT capable facilities and even fewer facilities willing to perform ECT in adolescents.

As is true for many treatments in child and adolescent psychiatry, there are few formal studies of ECT in adolescents.[3] Even facilities that are willing to perform ECT on adolescents may be hesitant to provide treatment for adolescents who have any potential contraindications. Although case reports have shown ECT to be safe in adolescents with inadequate nutrition (eg, patients with anorexia nervosa),[9] no studies to date have reported on safety of ECT for adolescents with a feeding tube.

The patient in this case, a 14-year-old girl, came to our hospital with symptoms consistent with catatonia. Through the course of her illness, she had stopped eating and had been living with a nasogastric tube in place for several weeks. On the recommendation of her local psychiatrist, her parents sought ECT treatment and found that multiple providers would not perform ECT because of her age, and others declined to provide the treatment because she had a nasogastric tube, with concerns for possible aspiration. She was accepted at Vanderbilt Psychiatric Hospital with plans to provide ECT.

CASE REPORT

The patient was a 14-year-old girl with a reported history of Kikuchi-Fujimoto disease who presented with signs of catatonia; she was noted only to intermittently follow commands but would not open her eyes, eat, or care for activities of daily living. At the time of admission, she had rarely spoken for several months and had a nasogastric tube in place owing to poor parenteral intake.

On hospital day 1, collateral information was gathered from physicians at an outside hospital. Previous treatment was discussed with the treating rheumatologist, the hospitalist on her primary team, and the hospitalist following her psychiatric care. She had been diagnosed with Kikuchi-Fujimoto disease 3 years before her admission to Vanderbilt. A few months before presentation, she developed headaches and was started on topiramate after failing other treatments. Shortly after beginning topiramate, she stopped eating and was admitted to a children's hospital near her home after showing signs of orthostatic hypotension.

At the outside hospital, a full gastrointestinal workup was done, and a nasogastric tube was placed. Rheumatology evaluated her for systemic lupus erythematosus and determined that she did not meet diagnostic criteria despite a positive anti-dsDNA. She was treated with pulse steroids with no improvement.

During her stay at the outside hospital, she showed signs and symptoms of depression and endorsed suicidal ideation. She was tried on escitalopram with worsening of symptoms. She began to show signs of catatonia and was tried on lorazepam without improvement. She was started on risperidone after endorsing auditory hallucinations. Risperidone was discontinued after she developed jaw stiffness. After 89 days, she was discharged home with a nasogastric tube with plans to follow up at a psychiatric hospital. She was admitted briefly to a local psychiatric hospital, but her parents withdrew her against medical advice after a few days. She returned home, where she gradually declined in function, and her catatonia progressed to the point where she would not speak, open her eyes, or make any purposeful movement.

When she presented to our hospital, her eyes were closed, she would intermittently respond to commands, and she would not speak. A lorazepam trial resulted in minimal benefit (dose was titrated to 2 mg orally every 6 hours). ECT was started on hospital day 5, with a Monday/Tuesday/Wednesday/Friday schedule. After the second ECT, she opened her eyes and began communicating. Throughout the first week of ECT, she was dysphoric, expressed passive suicidality, and was tearful and withdrawn throughout the day. She repeated her history almost word-for-word every day, focusing on somatic complaints, and minimizing psychiatric complaints. She continued to insist that the escitalopram caused her depression during her prior hospitalization. After her fourth ECT, she divulged to the treatment team that she had been sent sexually explicit pictures a few years prior, which resulted in cyber-bullying by kids at school. Since that time, she had struggled with depression and suicidal ideation, and had 2 unsuccessful suicide attempts. After her fifth ECT, the patient's affect brightened and she stated that she felt "good." She began to participate in group treatment, was able to walk on her own, and was consuming enough nutrition by mouth for the nasogastric tube to be removed. At this time, she began to minimize her symptoms and stated that she believed she got better because she wanted to, not because of the ECT. She continued with ECT and was discharged to the partial hospitalization program after her seventh treatment and a 19-day inpatient hospitalization, with plans to continue maintenance ECT. Throughout the hospitalization, the patient and family were resistant to starting medications, and no psychotropic medications were started. She completed a course of 9 total treatments and was referred to outpatient care in her home community. Throughout her hospital course, her parents spent a significant amount of time, energy, and money on travel and lodging, because they had to travel 225 miles from their home for treatment.

Each round of ECT was performed using a MECTA spECTrum 5000Q (MECTA Corporation, Portland, OR), with constant current delivery. Given the severity of her illness and lorazepam use, she was initially started on full-pulse bifrontotemporal/bilateral settings, which we continued throughout her treatment course. For each treatment, her settings were as follows:

Pulse width: 1 ms
Frequency: 60 Hz
Duration: 6 sec
Current: 800 mA
Charge: 576 mC

Our team monitored her ictal response through motor convulsive activity and electroencephalogram monitoring. Her typical electroencephalogram seizure duration ranged from 13 to 25 seconds, which was likely impacted by lorazepam dosing but offered a robust clinical response despite shorter duration.

Given her relative immobility for several weeks before her first treatment, only methohexital was used for the duration of her treatment course in an effort to avoid rapid potassium shifts. She was also given ketorolac tromethamine (Toradol) 30 mg intravenously ×1 with each treatment for pain management. She tolerated this treatment without pain or issues, so this dosing regimen was continued for all 9 treatments.

DISCUSSION

ECT has been shown to be a safe and effective treatment for many psychiatric disorders, and is especially effective for the treatment of catatonia regardless of the underlying cause; it has no absolute contraindications. However, the stigma surrounding this treatment remains, and providers are often cautious about and hesitant to administer ECT. This hesitancy has led to institutional policies against performing ECT in the context of potential relative contraindications. Although there is no clear evidence that ECT is unsafe in adolescents, there remain a limited number of providers or facilities that will treat patients under the age of 18. In additions, facilities that are able to administer treatment to adolescents are often cautious about treating patients with potential contraindications. In the case of our patient, the theoretic risk of aspiration became a barrier to appropriate care and placed a significant burden on the patient and family, who traveled 225 miles from their home for treatment.

When making the decision of whether or not to perform ECT, the risks and benefits of treatment should always be considered. For patients with persistent severe mental illness for which ECT is indicated, theoretic relative contraindications should not be treated as absolute contraindications. Without ECT, the patient's condition would likely have continued to deteriorate, putting her health at much greater risk than the potential risk of aspiration during treatment. This case has demonstrated that a feeding tube should not be treated as an absolute contraindication to ECT. As more evidence for the safety of ECT in adolescents being treated with a feeding tube is collected, medical facilities must adjust their policies to remove barriers to treatment.

REFERENCES

1. Payne NA, Prudic J. Electroconvulsive therapy part II: a biopsychosocial perspective. J Psychiatr Pract 2009;15(5):369–90.
2. American Psychiatric Association Task Force on ECT. ECT: methods of administration. In: Frankel FH, Bidder GT, Fink M, et al, editors. Electroconvulsive therapy (task force report # 14). Washington, DC: American Psychiatric Association; 1978. p. 92–121.

3. American Psychiatric Association Task Force on ECT. The practice of ECT: recommendations for treatment, training and privileging. Convuls Ther 1990;6(2):85–120.
4. Fink M, Shorter E, Taylor M. Catatonia is not schizophrenia: Kraepelin's error and the need to recognize catatonia as an independent syndrome in medical nomenclature. Schizophr Bull 2010;36(2):314–20.
5. Bica B, Moro A, Hax V, et al. Electroconvulsive therapy as a treatment for refractory neuropsychiatric lupus with catatonia: three case studies and literature review. Lupus 2015;24(12):1327–31.
6. Leon T, Aguirre A, Pesce C. Electroconvulsive therapy for catatonia in juvenile neuropsychiatric lupus. Lupus 2014;23(10):1066–8.
7. Aoki Y, Yamaguchi S, Ando S, et al. The experience of electroconvulsive therapy and its impact on associated stigma: a meta-analysis. Int J Soc Psychiatry 2016; 62(8):708–18.
8. Flamarique I, Baeza I, de la Serna E, et al. Thinking about electroconvulsive therapy: the opinions of parents of adolescents with schizophrenia spectrum disorders. J Child Adolesc Psychopharmacol 2017;27(1):75–82.
9. Andersen L, LaRosa C, Gih DE. Reexamining the role of electroconvulsive therapy in anorexia nervosa in adolescents. J ECT 2017;33(4):294–6.

Moving?

Make sure your subscription moves with you!

To notify us of your new address, find your **Clinics Account Number** (located on your mailing label above your name), and contact customer service at:

Email: journalscustomerservice-usa@elsevier.com

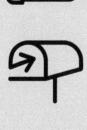

800-654-2452 (subscribers in the U.S. & Canada)
314-447-8871 (subscribers outside of the U.S. & Canada)

Fax number: 314-447-8029

Elsevier Health Sciences Division
Subscription Customer Service
3251 Riverport Lane
Maryland Heights, MO 63043

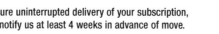